Dictionary
of Hearing

T0213514

Dictionary of Hearing

MICHAEL C. MARTIN OBE
The Mike Martin Consultancy

IAN R. SUMMERS
Medical Physics Group, School of Physics, University of Exeter

W

WHURR PUBLISHERS

LONDON

© 1999 Whurr Publishers
First published 1999 by
Whurr Publishers Ltd
19b Compton Terrace, London N1 2UN, England

Reprinted 2001

British Library Cataloguing in Publication Data
A catalogue record for this book is available from the
British Library.

ISBN: 1 86156 132 6

Introduction

Anyone who becomes interested in hearing will quickly discover that it is a particularly multidisciplinary subject. A topic in hearing may cross the fields of acoustics, audiology, electronics, medicine, phonetics, rehabilitation and/or social administration, to mention just a few. It is often difficult for someone whose background lies principally in only one of these fields to interpret relevant material that has a bias towards a less familiar discipline. This dictionary has been compiled with such problems in mind. The authors have included a wide range of terms that are in general use in the current literature on hearing and related topics. A selection of previously used but now outdated terms is also included, to assist in the interpretation of earlier literature.

In order to keep the dictionary to a manageable size, it has proved necessary to omit many terms relating to narrowly specialized medical and technical areas. Our principal rationale has been to cover the needs of the reader who is non-specialist in some relevant fields, of the lay person and of non-English speakers; (the needs of the specialist we hope will be supported by the availability of concise definitions of many terms in common usage). To some extent, however, the selection of terms reflects a personal choice on the part of the authors. Although having professional experience in many fields, the authors are probably most at home with technical topics and

there may be a slight bias towards these areas, making the dictionary particularly useful to the reader with a limited background in physics, acoustics or electronics, for example.

The International Electrotechnical Commission (IEC) has published defin-itions for many terms relating to hearing in their standard IEC 60050-801: International Electrotechnical Vocabulary·Chapter 801: Acoustics and electroacoustics, These defin-itions, where appropriate, have been included with the kind permission of the IEC. The terms with definitions taken from IEC 60050-801 include a reference to this standard, including the term number, abbreviated as IEC 801-22-22, for example. In some cases, indicated by 'modified' in the reference, the existing IEC definitions have been slightly modified for reasons of clarity. Similarly, terms with definitions taken from other standards are also fully referenced to their sources. Readers may wish to consult the IEC standard 60050-801, or the IEC compendium dictionary, for further definitions, relating to topics beyond those covered by this dictionary and also for translations into languages other than English.

Explanatory preface

Acronyms and similar letter combinations are listed alphabetically at the head of the letter sections, followed by other terms in alphabetical order. Where the term consists of more than one word, either with or without hyphens, its order in the alphabetical listing is determined primarily by the first word; for example, SIGN LANGUAGE is ahead of SIGNED ENGLISH.

The spelling in this dictionary is based upon the form of English used in the United Kingdom. In some cases the American-English spelling is also referred to, if this is sufficiently different to cause potential confusion, e.g., ETIOLOGY/AETIOLOGY.

At the end of a definition, indicated by 'See also .....', may be found a list of related terms defined elsewhere in the dictionary. However, such a list is non-inclusive: it features only terms that do not appear in the main text of the definition. The reader should bear in mind that terms used within the definition are often defined elsewhere in the dictionary – to avoid disrupting the text the authors have chosen not to indicate where this is the case.

Where appropriate, relevant technical standards are referred to by the initials of their originating organization (IEC, ISO, etc.) followed by the number of the standard, e.g., 'IEC 60318'. The full titles of these standards are given in Appendix 1 which also lists other standards that are relevant to the topics covered by the dictionary. The numbering of some standards has been changed recently: in such cases Appendix 1 indicates the previous as well as the current number.

Acknowledgements

The authors wish to acknowledge the considerable input from the late Professor D.W. Robinson of the Institute of Sound and Vibration Research, University of Southampton, UK, in reviewing and commenting on draft definitions. The authors are also indebted to Professor Stig Arlinger of the Department of Technical Audiology, University Hospital of Linköping, Sweden, for his helpful comments.

The permission of the IEC Central Office in Geneva to use terms from the IEC 60050-801 standard is gratefully acknowledged.

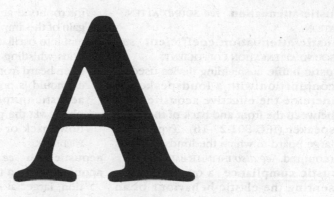

A-weighting the most commonly used of several frequency weightings (i.e., standardized frequency responses) incorporated in sound level meters. A-weighting is generally used when measuring industrial noise for hearing conservation purposes. It produces measurements that correlate reasonably well with subjective reactions to sound. Compared to a linear (i.e., flat) frequency response, A-weighting differs principally in terms of a marked reduction in response to frequencies below 500 Hz. The precise frequency response is detailed in IEC 651. *See* Figure 4, under FREQUENCY WEIGHTING.

ABLB test *see* ALTERNATE BINAURAL LOUDNESS-BALANCE TEST.

ABR *see* AUDITORY BRAINSTEM RESPONSE.

a.c. or AC originally serving only as an abbreviation for alternating current, the term is now also used in its own right to describe a fluctuating signal or signal component, generally with a mean value of zero.

AGC *see* AUTOMATIC GAIN CONTROL.

AM *see* AMPLITUDE MODULATION.

ANSI American National Standards Institute.

AP *see* ACTION POTENTIAL.

ART *see* ACOUSTIC-REFLEX THRESHOLD.

ASA American Standards Association.

ASHA American Speech Hearing and Language Association.

ASL or ASLAN American sign language. *see* SIGN LANGUAGE.

AVC *see* AUTOMATIC VOLUME CONTROL.

absolute pitch the attribute of a person who can judge the pitch of a musical note accurately and/or can accurately produce a note of a certain pitch on demand, without needing a reference against which pitch comparisons can be made. Also known as perfect pitch. *See also* RELATIVE PITCH.

absorption *see* SOUND ABSORPTION.

absorption coefficient *see* SOUND ABSORPTION COEFFICIENT.

acceleration the rate of change of velocity.

accelerometer a transducer which produces an electrical output proportional to the acceleration of the object to which it is secured. Accelerometers are used routinely to measure the motion of vibrating surfaces.

accommodation *see* ADAPTATION.

acoustic absorption *see* SOUND ABSORPTION.

acoustic absorption coefficient *see* SOUND ABSORPTION COEFFICIENT.

acoustic admittance at a given surface, the reciprocal of the acoustic impedance at the surface. The accepted symbol is Y.

acoustic aid a hearing aid that relies purely upon an acoustic system to provide amplification or to transmit sound from one place to another, e.g., an ear trumpet, a speaking tube.

acoustic attenuation *see* SOUND ATTENUATION.

acoustic attenuation coefficient *see* SOUND ATTENUATION COEFFICIENT.

acoustic baffle a shielding device used in conjunction with a loudspeaker to increase the effective acoustic path between the front and back of the loudspeaker (IEC 801-27-16). Typically a large board in which the loudspeaker is mounted. *See also* INFINITE BAFFLE.

acoustic compliance a quantity representing the elastic behaviour of an acoustic system. In a system whose behaviour is dominated by elastic effects, the acoustic compliance at a given surface is equal to the volume displacement divided by the sound pressure. An acoustic compliance C_A contributes a term of magnitude $1/2\pi f C_A$ to the acoustic impedance at frequency f. The acoustic compliance at the input surface of a system, such as the eardrum at the input of the middle ear, represents the ease with which the input surface can be moved by an external pressure.

acoustic coupler (1) a cavity of specified shape and volume which is used for the calibration of an earphone in conjunction with a calibrated microphone to measure the sound pressure developed within the cavity (IEC 303). Acoustic couplers have cavities varying in size according to their use, e.g., the *6 cc coupler* (IEC 303) is used with supra-aural earphones while the *2 cc coupler* (IEC 126) is used for hearing-aid insert earphones. In contrast to artificial ears, acoustic couplers do not attempt to represent accurately the acoustic impedance of the human ear. *See also* EAR SIMULATOR.

acoustic coupler (2) a device to connect a telephone handset to a modem or terminal for acoustical transfer of digital data.

acoustic feedback the passage of sound from an earphone, loudspeaker etc. at the output of an amplifying system to a microphone at its input. Owing to the gain of the amplifier this may set the system into oscillation, producing a continuous whistling sound. This whistling is often heard from hearing aids where the earmould is poorly fitting, allowing the acoustic output to reach the microphone via the poor seal. Also known as howl back or howl around. *See also* FEEDBACK.

acoustic gain *see* AIR-TO-AIR GAIN.

acoustic horn a tube of varying cross section, larger at one end than the other, intended to achieve an acoustic impedance match and, possibly, to produce a directional effect (IEC 801-27-12).

acoustic immittance a generic term covering a range of terms related to acoustic impedance and admittance, such as acoustic impedance, acoustic admittance, acoustic compliance, acoustic resistance, etc.

acoustic impedance at a given surface, the complex quotient of sound pressure p, averaged over the surface, and the volume velocity U through it. The accepted symbol for acoustic impedance is Z, i.e. $Z = p/U$, and the unit is the pascal second per metre cubed (Pa s m^{-3}). The quantity usually measured is the modulus of the complex quantity defined above (IEC 1027). *See also* ACOUSTIC COMPLIANCE, ACOUSTIC RESISTANCE, INERTANCE, MECHANICAL IMPEDANCE.

acoustic-impedance audiometry *see* TYMPANOMETRY.

acoustic inertance *see* INERTANCE.

acoustic insulation *see* SOUND INSULATION.

acoustic intensity *see* SOUND INTENSITY.

acoustic mass *see* INERTANCE.

acoustic meatus *see* EAR CANAL, INTERNAL AUDITORY MEATUS.

acoustic medium a medium within which sound waves can propagate.

acoustic nerve *see* AUDITORY NERVE.

acoustic neuroma a tumour on the auditory nerve.

acoustic phonetics the branch of linguistics that deals with speech sounds, i.e., their acoustic nature and the manner in which they are produced.

acoustic pressure *see* SOUND PRESSURE.

acoustic reflex a contraction of the stapedius muscle in the middle ear in response to an acoustic stimulus. This causes tensioning of the eardrum, thus reducing the transmission of sound through the middle ear. The reflex is normally bilateral. Also called aural reflex, middle-ear reflex or stapedius reflex.

acoustic-reflex threshold (ART) of an ear and for a specified type of sound, the lowest level of that sound which elicits the acoustic reflex. The ART is commonly expressed in terms of hearing level.

acoustic resistance the component of acoustic impedance corresponding to resistive behaviour. In a system whose behaviour is dominated by resistive effects, the acoustic resistance at a given surface is equal to the sound pressure divided by the volume velocity. *See also* MECHANICAL RESISTANCE.

acoustic shock a term used in telephony to describe a sudden loud sound from a telephone earpiece. To prevent damage to the ear, a level of 118 dB SPL is often used by telecommunications standards bodies as the maximum output from a telephone earpiece.

acoustic test box a box which has been acoustically treated so that it is non-reverberant and in which sounds at calibrated sound pressure levels can be generated. Used to evaluate the electro-acoustic performance of devices such as microphones, hearing aids, etc. Also known simply as a test box.

acoustic trauma sudden damage to hearing caused by loud sound, in particular loud impulsive sound. This term is normally reserved for damage produced by a single event, as opposed to long-term cumulative hearing loss.

acoustic tubing tubing that is used to convey an acoustic signal from one point to another. The term is widely used to denote the tubing that carries the acoustic signal from a behind-the-ear hearing aid to the earmould.

acoustician a person specializing in some aspect of acoustics.

acoustics the science of the production, control, transmission, reception and effects of sound.

acquired hearing loss a hearing loss that the hearing-impaired person was not born with. The term is usually used in relation to adults who have become hearing impaired in later life.

action potential (AP) a self-propagating wave of electric potential which travels along a nerve cell as a consequence of the cell being stimulated.

active electrode an electrode used for stimulation or measurement whose electric potential is determined with respect to a second electrode, the indifferent or reference electrode, at zero potential.

active filter a frequency-selective system whose response is determined partly by components which draw on an external power source. The basilar membrane is an example; its response is partly determined by mechanical input from the outer hair cells.

active transducer a transducer in which the energy of the output signal is derived, at least in part, from sources other than the input signal (IEC 801-25-06 modified). For example, a microphone which includes a battery-powered amplifier. *See also* PASSIVE TRANSDUCER.

acute (1) in the sense of *acute illness*, a term used to describe an illness which comes sharply to a crisis. The opposite of chronic, which implies a long-standing condition.

acute (2) in the sense of *acute hearing*, a term used to describe hearing which is more sensitive than normal.

adaptation a decrease in the output of sensory receptors in response to a constant signal. In hearing this leads to a drop in sensitivity of the ear when it is subjected to a continuous sound. Also known as accommodation. *See also* AUDITORY FATIGUE, HABITUATION, TONE DECAY.

adaptive test a test in which the test signals presented to the subject vary according to the previous responses the subject has made. For instance, if the subject does not respond to a sound stimulus because it is too quiet, the loudness of the stimulus is automatically increased by the test equipment until the subject responds; if the subject responds appropriately on a consistent basis, the stimulus is made quieter. Adaptive test procedures are efficient in the sense that they ensure that most test material is neither too easy nor too difficult for the subject.

admittance *see* ACOUSTIC ADMITTANCE.

aerodynamic noise *see* HYDRODYNAMIC NOISE.

aetiology (of a disease) the origin or causes of a disease. The American spelling is etiology.

afferent nerve a nerve which conducts signals from peripheral organs to the central nervous system. *See also* EFFERENT NERVE

affricate a speech sound which combines a plosive with a fricative in a rapid sequence, e.g., *ch* as in chair. *See also* MANNER OF ARTICULATION.

age-associated hearing loss *see* PRESBY-ACUSIS.

aid *see* HEARING AID.

air-bone gap of an ear, the hearing threshold level measured by air conduction minus the hearing threshold level measured by bone conduction. A significant positive air-bone gap suggests malfunction of the outer or middle ear.

air conduction transmission of sound through the outer and middle ear to the inner ear (ISO 8253-1).

air-to-air gain the gain of an acoustic amplifying system. For a hearing aid, the difference between the sound pressure level developed in an acoustic coupler or ear simulator by the output from the hearing aid and the corresponding sound pressure level measured at the input test point. Also known as acoustic gain. *See also* IN-SITU GAIN.

alternate binaural loudness-balance test (ABLB test) a procedure in which the loudness of a signal in one ear is balanced against the loudness of a signal in the other ear, the two signals being presented alternately. This test can be used to determine if abnormal perception of loudness, i.e., recruitment, is present in cases of hearing loss.

alternative augmentative communication forms of communication offered to people who cannot speak, whose speech is unintelligible or who have problems in finding words. The techniques used range from signing and simple pointing boards to computerized systems that allow speech to be produced artificially.

alveolar a term used in the classification of consonants, describing the position of the tongue when it comes into contact with the alveolar ridge behind the teeth during the production of a consonant.

ambient noise background noise in the area of a listener or where acoustical measurements are being made, usually a composite of sounds from many sources, near and far. *See also* SOCIAL NOISE.

amplification the increase in amplitude or power of a signal, usually by electronic means.

amplified telephone a telephone with a built-in amplifier to provide a louder received signal at the earpiece. The term may also be used to describe a telephone that provides amplification for the outgoing speech signal.

amplifier a device, usually electronic, that increases the amplitude or power of a signal.

amplitude the 'size' of a signal, usually defined in terms of the magnitude of signal excursions from some zero level or equilibrium condition. Different measures can be used, for example peak amplitude (the maximum signal excursion), peak-to-peak amplitude (the difference between the most negative and most positive excursions), root-mean-square amplitude (an average value of signal excursions over time). *See also* PEAK-TO-PEAK-EQUIVALENT SOUND PRESSURE LEVEL.

amplitude compression *see* COMPRESSION.

amplitude distribution a method of representing a time-varying signal by indicating the percentage of time that the signal level occupies each of a series of amplitude intervals. Also known as cumulative distribution.

amplitude envelope a line joining successive peaks (either all positive or all negative) of a time-varying signal, which indicates how the amplitude of the signal varies with time.

amplitude modulation (AM) variation of the amplitude of a constant-frequency carrier signal in such a way that the resulting amplitude envelope has the form of a particular lower-frequency signal (the modulating signal). For example, in AM radio, the amplitude of a carrier signal of frequency 1 MHz, say, is modulated by a speech or music signal in the audio-frequency range.

amplitude response of a system such as an electronic amplifier or filter, for a given input frequency, the ratio of the output amplitude to the input amplitude (i.e. the gain of the system at that frequency). The amplitude response can be measured over a range of frequencies and plotted as a function of frequency, in which case the resulting graph is referred to as the frequency response of the system. *See also* TRANSFER FUNCTION, PHASE RESPONSE.

analogue device a device, typically an electronic system, in which a continuously variable signal is represented in its original form – as a continuously varying voltage, for example (as opposed to a digital device in which signals are represented as binary information, coded as transitions between two discrete states).

analogue display a display with an indication via a moving pointer on a scale or dial, as opposed to a digital display, which has a direct indication by means of figures.

anechoic without echoes.

anechoic chamber *see* ANECHOIC ROOM.

anechoic room a room without echoes or reverberation whose boundaries effectively absorb all incident sound over the frequency range of interest, thereby creating an essentially free sound field in a specified test space. Mainly used for acoustic testing of loudspeakers, microphones, etc. Also known as an anechoic chamber or free-field room. *See also* DEAD ROOM.

antenatal in the period before the birth of a child. *See also* PERINATAL, POSTNATAL.

antinode a point, line or surface in a standing wave where some specified characteristic of the wave field has maximum amplitude (IEC 801-23-17). *See also* NODE.

anti-noise sound directed into a given region in such a manner and with such a waveform as to cancel or partially cancel the sound previously existing in that region, for the purposes of noise reduction.

anti-noise microphone *see* NOISE-CANCELLING MICROPHONE.

antiphase the relation between two similar signals of opposite phase, i.e., of similar waveform but one inverted with respect to the other.

antiresonance in a system which is driven to oscillate, a phenomenon which produces a minimum response at a particular frequency (the anti-resonant frequency). The converse of resonance, which produces a maximum response.

antitragus *see* TRAGUS.

aperiodic a term used to describe a signal whose features do not repeat. *See also* PERIODIC.

aphasia a condition which causes a partial or total loss of the ability to use or to understand language, following damage to the brain.

articulation movements of the vocal tract to produce speech.

articulation function *see* SPEECH RECOGNITION CURVE.

articulation score (1) a term formerly used in audiology to denote the percentage of speech units correctly identified out of a test list. This term is no longer recommended by ISO and has been replaced by the term speech recognition score, see ISO 8253-3.

articulation score (2) a term used in speech therapy to denote the percentage of speech sounds produced correctly.

artificial ear a device for the calibration of an earphone which presents to the earphone an acoustic impedance equivalent to the impedance presented by the average human ear. It is equipped with a calibrated microphone for the measurement of the sound pressure developed by the earphone. Also known as an ear simulator (this latter term is now also used as a generic term for both acoustic coupler and artificial ear). *See also* ACOUSTIC COUPLER, OCCLUDED-EAR SIMULATOR.

artificial head and torso *see* HEAD AND TORSO SIMULATOR.

artificial larynx a device used by persons who have had their larynx removed. It generates a sound in the mouth similar to that produced by the vocal cords in normal speech. The sound is fed into the mouth either from a vibrator placed on the throat or from a tube entering the mouth, allowing speech production by modulating this sound in the normal manner, i.e., as if the sound were being generated by the larynx.

artificial manikin *see* HEAD AND TORSO SIMULATOR.

artificial mastoid a device for measurement of the output from the bone vibrators which are used with audiometers and hearing aids. It provides a mechanical load that closely approximates the mechanical impedance of the average human mastoid process, and incorporates a mechano-electrical transducer to measure the vibratory force or acceleration generated by the bone vibrator. A close approximation to the mechanical impedance of the human mastoid process is very difficult to realize. Hence, in practice, the output of bone vibrators is measured using a mechanical coupler, described in IEC 60318-6, which provides a specified mechanical load – not an exact match to the mastoid process but of the right order.

artificial mouth a device consisting of a loudspeaker unit mounted in a baffle or an enclosure so shaped as to have an acoustic radiation pattern similar to that of the average human mouth. (IEC 801-28-06).

artificial voice a complex sound, usually emitted by an artificial mouth, whose spectrum corresponds to that of the average human voice (IEC 801-28-07). An artificial mouth emitting an artificial voice may be referred to as a voice simulator.

assistive device a device used by a deaf or hard-of-hearing person to give awareness of an acoustic signal, usually a warning signal such as a door bell, fire alarm, etc. For example, making use of a flashing-light indicator.

assistive listening device an amplifying device, other than a hearing aid, for use by a hard-of-hearing person, e.g., a TV listening aid, induction-loop system or infrared transmission system.

asymmetrical hearing loss a hearing loss in which the individual losses of each ear are significantly different.

atresia a narrowing or closing of a vessel or organ.

attack time in an AGC system, the time taken for the circuit to respond to a sudden increase of input level, i.e. the time taken to bring down the output level to the appropriate value. *See also* RELEASE TIME.

attenuation the reduction in level of a signal. *See also* SOUND ATTENUATION.

attenuation coefficient *see* SOUND ATTENUATION COEFFICIENT.

attenuator a device for reducing the level

of a signal in calibrated steps, these steps being usually equal when expressed in decibels. Laboratory attenuators will often have 0.1, 1 and 10 dB steps to allow for fine control of signal level. Audiometers usually have 5 dB steps on the hearing-level control, which is an attenuator operating on the output signal.

audible sound (1) an acoustic oscillation of such character as to be capable of exciting a sensation of hearing (IEC 801-21-02a).

audible sound (2) a sensation of hearing

evoked by an acoustic oscillation or vibration (IEC 801-21-02b modified). Often simply referred to as a sound.

audio frequency a frequency in the range that is audible, usually taken to be 20 to 20,000 Hz, but quoted by some authorities as 16 to 16,000 Hz.

audio-visual speech perception the perception of speech using both the acoustic speech signal and visual information from observation of the lips and other movements of the speaker. *See also* LIP READING.

audiogram (1) *pure-tone audiogram*: a

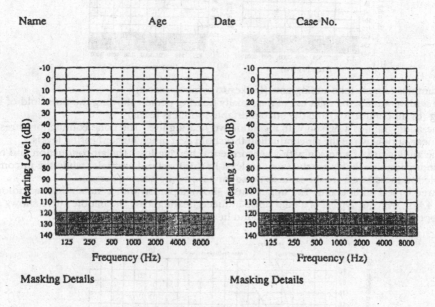

PURE TONE AUDIOGRAM

Name   Age   Date   Case No.

Masking Details   Masking Details

	Right	Left
Air conduction, masked if necessary	O	X
Air conduction, not masked (shadow point)	●	X
Bone conduction, not masked	Δ	
Bone conduction, masked	[	]
Uncomfortable loudness level	L	⌐

Figure 1.

a) Typical format for a pure-tone audiogram as recommended by the British Society of Audiology (BSA 1975) and in keeping with the recommendations in ISO 8253-1.

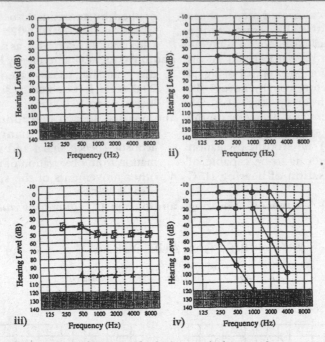

i) ii)

iii) iv)

b) Examples of pure-tone audiograms [for key to symbols, see a)]:
i) An audiogram for the right ear of a normally hearing person showing the threshold of hearing (by air-conduction) and the uncomfortable loudness levels.
ii) The audiogram of a person with a conductive hearing loss. The bone conduction threshold is near normal while the air-conduction threshold is at much higher hearing levels.
iii) The audiogram of a person with a sensorineural hearing loss. The air-conduction and bone-conduction thresholds are the same (at least in this idealized example) while the uncomfortable loudness levels are the same as those for a normally hearing person.
iv) Three typical audiograms: The upper curve shows a person with a 'notch' in the audiogram at 4 kHz which is typical of a mild noise-induced hearing loss. The middle curve shows a ski-slope loss and the lower curve a profound hearing loss or 'corner audiogram'.

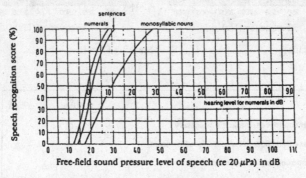

c) The format for a speech audiogram. The x-axis in this example, for use with speech signals being produced by a loudspeaker, is in terms of sound pressure level. The three curves on the audiogram are reference speech recognition curves for different types of test material. The supplementary horizontal axis, half-way up the frame, indicates hearing level for the test material consisting of numerals. (From Brinkmann and Richter 1997)

Figure 1. (contd)

10

chart depicting the threshold of hearing of an individual as measured by a pure-tone audiometer at a number of frequencies across the range 125 to 8000 Hz. High-frequency audiometry extends the audiogram up to 16 kHz. The threshold is measured in decibels, with zero on the scale (audiometric zero) being based on the modal value of the threshold of hearing for young adults in the age range 18 to 30 years. *See* Figure 1 a), b).

audiogram (2) *speech audiogram*: a chart showing the ability of a person to understand speech (using specially prepared test material) as a function of the loudness of the speech. The test is scored in terms of the percentage of words or phonemes correctly recognized. *See* Figure 1 c.

audiological physician an appropriately qualified physician who practises in audiology.

audiological scientist an appropriately qualified scientist who practises in audiology.

audiologist a person who practises audiology. Normally someone who is concerned with the prevention of hearing loss and/or the detection, diagnosis and rehabilitation of adults or children with hearing loss.

audiology the science of hearing. *See also* CLINICAL AUDIOLOGY.

audiology technician a person who has recognized training and who practices audiology under medical supervision.

audiometer (1) an electroacoustic instrument for the measurement of hearing, most commonly for measuring the hearing threshold level.

audiometer (2) *automatic-recording audiometer*: an audiometer in which signal presentations, frequency selection or variation, hearing level variation, and the recording of the subject's responses are implemented automatically. The direction of hearing level changes is under the subject's control. An automatic recording audiometer may have facilities for presenting fixed frequencies or a continuously variable (sweep) frequency, or both; it may also provide both continuous and pulsed tone outputs. Also called a self-recording audiometer. *See also* BÉKÉSY AUDIOMETRY.

audiometer (3) *computer-controlled audiometer*: an audiometer in which the test procedure is controlled by a computer or microprocessor. Often the calculation and display of hearing threshold levels, derived from the subject's responses, are also implemented.

audiometer (4) *manual audiometer*: an audiometer in which the signal presentations, frequency and hearing level selection, and the noting of the subject's responses, are performed manually.

audiometer (5) *pure-tone audiometer*: an audiometer equipped (for air conduction measurements) with earphones and headband, which provides pure tones of specified frequencies at known sound pressure levels, one ear at a time. For bone conduction measurements, the audiometer is also equipped with a bone vibrator. For clinical use, both facilities are required, as well as means of generating calibrated masking noise. An external-input port is usually provided for connection to an external signal source.

audiometer (6) *speech audiometer*: an electroacoustic instrument for the measurement of hearing using speech test material. A pure-tone audiometer often has the means to be used as a speech audiometer by connecting a source of pre-recorded speech material to the external-input port.

audiometric booth a small cabin, usually taking one person seated, intended for the testing of hearing. *See also* AUDIOMETRIC ROOM.

audiometric descriptor a subjective description given to hearing threshold levels depicted on an audiogram, e.g., mild hearing loss, moderate hearing loss, severe hearing loss, profound hearing loss.

The British Society of Audiology recommendation (BSA 1988) for audiometric descriptors is as follows:

Audiometric descriptor	dB HL
Mild hearing loss	20–40
Moderate hearing loss	41–70
Severe hearing loss	71–95
Profound hearing loss	> 95

The hearing level values (HL) are based on the average of the pure tone threshold levels at 250, 500, 1000, 2000 and 4000 Hz.

audiometric frequencies those frequencies standardized for use with pure-tone audiometers, i.e., 125, 250, 500, 750, 1000, 1500, 2000, 3000, 4000, 6000, 8000 Hz . Audiometers for use in the extended high-frequency range use frequencies from the following: 8000, 9000, 10,000, 11,200, 12,500, 14,000, 16,000 Hz.

audiometric room a room insulated against outside noise and having some sound absorption, intended for testing hearing. (IEC 801-31-20). Quiet conditions are necessary to test hearing, particularly for testing those with near-normal hearing, as the detection of very faint sounds is generally involved.

audiometric zero the set of signal levels, for pure tones at audiometric frequencies, with respect to which hearing level and hearing threshold level are measured. Audiometric zero is specified for air conduction, in terms of the reference equivalent threshold sound pressure level (RETSPL), and for bone conduction, in terms of the reference equivalent threshold force level (RETFL). It corresponds to the 0 dB HL line on a pure-tone audiogram. *See also* MINIMUM AUDIBLE FIELD, RETSPL, RETFL.

audiometrician an alternative term for audiology technician.

audiometrist a person qualified to undertake routine audiometry.

audiometry the process of measuring the hearing of an individual, usually the threshold of hearing, using an audio-meter. This term is also used in a general sense to mean any measurement of the hearing system. *See also* HIGH-FREQUENCY AUDIOMETRY, PURE-TONE AUDIOMETRY, SPEECH AUDIOMETRY.

auditory relating to hearing.

auditory brainstem response (ABR) an electrical signal generated by the activity of the brainstem in response to an acoustic signal at the ear, i.e., the component of the auditory evoked response which derives from the activity of the brainstem. This response is used in ABR audiometry to measure the functioning of the brainstem.

auditory cortex that part of the brain that is particularly concerned with hearing.

auditory critical band *see* CRITICAL BAND.

auditory evoked potential *see* AUDITORY EVOKED RESPONSE.

auditory evoked response an electrical signal generated by the activity of the auditory nervous system in response to an acoustic signal at the ear. The signal, detected via scalp electrodes, can be measured only using computer averaging and signal processing techniques. Also known as auditory evoked potential.

auditory-evoked-response audiometry audiometry in which the electrical activity of the auditory nervous system, in response to tone bursts or clicks, is determined from measurements via scalp electrodes. Signal averaging over multiple stimulations is used to enhance the waveform and reduce the effect of other electrical activity. Also known as evoked-response audiometry (ERA) and electric-response audiometry (ERA). *See also* CORTICAL-EVOKED-RESPONSE AUDIOMETRY, ELECTROCOCHLEOGRAPHY.

auditory fatigue an alternative term for adaptation, but used mainly with reference to constant stimulation by a strong signal. *See also* HABITUATION.

auditory feedback a term used to describe hearing one's own voice.

auditory filter one of the large, overlapping set of bandpass filters which can be used to represent filtering within the auditory system, i.e., the process by which an acoustic input is decomposed into components at different frequencies. This filtering is largely associated with the hair cells and related structures.

auditory localization the ability to locate the direction from which a sound is coming, making use of differences in intensity and/or phase between the two ears. Also known as directional hearing. *See also* LATERALIZATION.

auditory meatus *see* EAR CANAL, INTERNAL AUDITORY MEATUS.

auditory nerve the nerve which takes neural signals from the cochlea to the brainstem. Sometimes called the acoustic nerve, the cochlear nerve, the eighth cranial nerve or the VIIIth nerve.

auditory-oral (approach to deaf education) *see* ORALISM.

auditory ossicles *see* OSSICLES.

auditory pathways the neural pathways that take the signals from the cochlea to the auditory cortex.

auditory periphery *see* PERIPHERAL AUDITORY SYSTEM.

auditory rehabilitation the process by which a person who has a hearing loss is taught to use his/her residual hearing.

auditory-response cradle a device in which infants are placed to measure their ability to hear. Physiological measurements are made in response to the presentation of acoustic signals.

auditory sensation area the region enclosed by the curves defining the threshold of hearing and the threshold of pain as functions of frequency (IEC 801-29-27).

auditory threshold *see* THRESHOLD OF HEARING.

auditory training unit a device used mainly in the education of deaf children. It consists of a microphone, an amplifier with one or more controls, and large earphones to enable a high acoustic output to be achieved over a wide frequency range, i.e., to achieve a better performance than a wearable hearing aid. Also called a speech trainer or auditory trainer.

auditory tube *see* EUSTACHIAN TUBE.

aural relating to the ear.

aural harmonic a harmonic of a periodic sound stimulus which is generated in the auditory system and perceived by the listener (IEC 801-29-39 modified).

aural-oral approach an educational approach used with deaf children which relies heavily on hearing, using amplification, and using the spoken word.

aural reflex *see* ACOUSTIC REFLEX.

auricle (1) the visible part of the outer ear, also called the pinna.

auricle (2) an acoustic aid which has the appearance of a horn mounted on the side of the head.

auriscope *see* OTOSCOPE.

automatic gain control (AGC) a means, in an amplifier, by which the gain is automatically controlled as a function of the magnitude of the envelope of the input signal or other signal parameter (IEC 118-2). In a hearing aid, an AGC circuit may be used to implement compression of signals, i.e., to reduce the dynamic range of the output compared to that of the input. *See also* AUTOMATIC VOLUME CONTROL.

automatic-recording audiometer *see* AUDIOMETER (2).

automatic-recording audiometry measurement of hearing with an automatic-recording audiometer. *See also* AUDIO-METER (2).

automatic speech recognition (ASR) the recognition of speech by a computer system.

automatic volume control (AVC) a general term for the means by which the maximum output of an amplifier is limited. In a hearing aid, AVC is generally implemented with an automatic gain control or by using peak clipping.

autophonic scale a scale which relates a speaker's estimate of his/her voice level to the measured sound pressure level of the voice.

B

B-weighting a standardized frequency weighting for sound level meters, now obsolete. *See* Figure 4, under FREQUENCY WEIGHTING.

BFO *see* BEAT-FREQUENCY OSCILLATOR.

BICROS *see* CROS.

BSL British sign language. *See* SIGN LANGUAGE.

BTE aid *see* BEHIND-THE-EAR AID.

background noise noise that is not central to what is being measured or listened to. The noise may be acoustic or generated as electrical noise in the measuring or sound-reproduction equipment. *See also* AMBIENT NOISE.

backward masking a phenomenon whereby the detectability of a signal is reduced in the period just preceding the onset of a masking noise. Also known as pre-stimulatory masking. *See also* FORWARD MASKING.

baffle *see* ACOUSTIC BAFFLE.

balance *see* SOUND BALANCE, VESTIBULAR SYSTEM.

balanced input an electrical input port is said to be balanced when the two input terminals have the same value of internal impedance with respect to a reference point and are intended to receive signals which are equal in magnitude but of opposite polarity with respect to that point (IEC 268-2 modified.). Balanced inputs have the advantage of minimizing stray signals picked up on the incoming signal cable and are used where cables are long and the input signals are weak.

bandpass filter or **band-pass filter** a filter which passes only those signals which lie within a specified range of frequencies. The frequency range, i.e., the bandwidth of the filter, is often specified in octaves or 1/3 octaves, but may also be specified in hertz (Hz) or as a percentage of the filter centre frequency.

bandstop filter or **band-stop filter** a filter which passes only those signals which lie outside a specified range of frequencies.

bandwidth (1) of a device, the frequency range over which the device operates in a specified manner. The bandwidth of a filter or linear amplifier is usually specified in terms of upper and lower cut-off frequencies at which the response has fallen by 3 dB from a nominal value. The bandwidth of a hearing aid is specified in terms of the frequencies at which the response of the aid has fallen by 20 dB from the average of the gains at 1000, 1600 and 2500 Hz.

bandwidth (2) of a signal, the frequency range which includes all significant frequency components of the signal.

bar chart a graphic representation of data, consisting of a series of vertical bars whose lengths indicate the magnitudes of the quantities represented.

Bárány box a clockwork-powered mechanical noise source which produces a rasping sound, used as a source of masking signal in the early days of audiometry.

Bárány chair a rotating chair used in the investigation of vestibular problems.

bark scale a distorted frequency scale on which the widths of the auditory critical bands are equal. (In the conventional frequency scale, critical bands at higher frequencies are wider than those at lower frequencies – this variation in bandwidth is eliminated by distortion of the conventional scale into a bark scale.) The unit on this scale is the bark: one bark is the width of each critical band. It is possible to construct similar scales based on other measures of the auditory-filter bandwidth.

barotrauma the injurious effect on the hearing and vestibular system of an increase in pressure. Conditions where the air pressure is outside the normal range of atmospheric values, such as underwater diving, may lead to barotrauma.

barrier microphone *see* BOUNDARY MICROPHONE.

basal forming the base, e.g., the basal turn of the cochlea.

basic frequency response the frequency response of a device which is considered to best represent its performance. Specifically, in hearing aids, the frequency response obtained with a 60 dB SPL input at the reference gain setting. *See also* COMPREHENSIVE FREQUENCY RESPONSE.

basilar membrane a membrane upon which lie the hair cells, forming part of the cochlear partition which divides the cross-section of the cochlea in two. *See* Figure 2, under EAR.

bass (in acoustics) low frequency sound.

bass boost a term used to label the tone control on an audio amplifier, indicating that low frequencies in the output are increased (i.e., boosted) by this control. *See also* BASS CUT, HIGH-FREQUENCY BOOST, HIGH-FREQUENCY CUT.

bass cut a term used to label the tone con-

trol on an audio amplifier, indicating that low frequencies in the output are decreased (i.e., cut) by this control. *See also* BASS BOOST, HIGH-FREQUENCY BOOST, HIGH-FREQUENCY CUT.

bass-reflex speaker a loudspeaker system, i.e., a loudspeaker in an acoustic enclosure, with a particular design that gives enhanced acoustic output at low frequencies. The enclosure allows radiation of the low-frequency sound emitted from the rear surface of the loudspeaker cone as well as that emitted from the front surface.

battery strictly speaking, an assembly of electrical cells which can provide a source of DC electricity. However, the term is generally applied to a single cell, one or more of which is used, for example, in an electric torch. *See also* TEST BATTERY.

battery current the current that a device takes from a battery. A given battery will have a specified maximum current for proper use and maximum life. Also known as battery drain or battery drain current. *See also* QUIESCENT CURRENT.

battery drain *see* BATTERY CURRENT.

battery of tests *see* TEST BATTERY.

baud rate the speed at which information is transmitted through a telecommunications or computer system. The unit is the baud, corresponding to one information-carrying pulse per second.

baudot a term used to describe a 5-bit mode of data transmission used in telegraphy, commonly used in the USA and some other countries with text telephones for deaf people.

beat(s) a phenomenon that results from the superposition of two waves whose frequencies are close to one another. For two such sounds at audible frequencies, a variation of loudness is heard at a low frequency known as the beat frequency, equal to the difference between the frequencies of the two superposed waves. If the beat frequency is reduced to zero by adjusting the two superposed waves to have identical frequencies, this is known as the zero-beat condition.

beat frequency *see* BEAT.

beat-frequency oscillator (BFO) an oscillator whose output frequency is derived from the beats between a variable-frequency signal and a fixed-frequency signal, using a heterodyne system. The term is also used in radio applications to describe a source of fixed-frequency signal, used to beat with received signals.

behavioural test a test which requires an active response from the person or animal being tested.

behind-the-ear aid (BTE aid) a hearing aid with all the components, except the earmould, in a case worn behind the ear. Also called a post-aural or post-auricular aid.

Békésy audiometry a form of automatic-recording audiometry, originally devised by Georg von Békésy, in which the test signal is a glide tone, i.e., with a continuously swept frequency, which the subject is intended to maintain at or near threshold. The term has sometimes been used as synonymous with automatic-recording audiometry, but is recommended to be reserved for automatic-recording audiometry with a continuous frequency sweep, as distinguished from fixed-frequency automatic-recording audiometry.

bel a unit for the measurement of amplitude, power or intensity, named after Alexander Graham Bell. The decibel, one tenth of a bel, is always used in practice. *See* DECIBEL.

Bell's palsy a facial paralysis produced by a disorder of the facial nerve.

bending wave a transverse wave in a plate or bar, being a combination of compressional and shear wave (IEC 801-23-11).

bilabial a description of the production of certain speech sounds, indicating that both lips are placed together, e.g., the sounds *p*, *b* and *m*.

bilateral relating to both sides of a structure, e.g., when both ears are receiving signals there is said to be bilateral stimulation. *See also* UNILATERAL.

bilingual the ability of an individual to communicate in two different languages with the proficiency of a native speaker in each language.

binaural involving the use of both ears for listening.

binaural advantage the increase of sensitivity or selectivity which results from listening with two ears rather than one.

binaural beats a phenomenon by which beats may be heard by the listener between two signals presented separately to each ear, produced by an interaction in the nervous system of the neural outputs from each ear.

binaural integration the combination of information from each ear to produce an enhanced perception compared to that available from either of the individual-ear signals.

binaural loudness balance *see* LOUDNESS BALANCE.

binaural loudness-balance test *see* ALTERNATE BINAURAL LOUDNESS-BALANCE TEST.

binaural summation the combination of information from each ear to produce a perception corresponding to the sum of the individual-ear signals.

Bing test a test for conductive deafness using a tuning fork, which involves closing the ear canal with a finger. For subjects without middle-ear impairment, this increases the sensitivity to bone-conduction signals at frequencies below 1 kHz. For subjects with significant middle-ear impairment, plugging the canal has no effect. *See also* RINNE TEST, TUNING-FORK TESTS, WEBER TEST.

biphasic pulse a short-duration signal during which the current (or voltage, etc.) is first positive and then negative, or vice versa. Biphasic electrical pulses may be used for nerve stimulation, in which case the positive and negative components are generally balanced to give no net flow of charge. Also known as a bipolar pulse. *See also* MONOPHASIC PULSE.

bipolar pulse *see* BIPHASIC PULSE.

bit binary digit, i.e., a 1 or a 0, the basis of digital information.

blind-deaf *see* DEAF-BLIND.

bodyworn aid or **body-worn aid** a hearing aid whose controls, amplifier and battery are contained in a case which is worn on the body, in a pocket or on the clothing . The earphone is connected by a lead or cord from the case of the aid. Known as a pocket aid in the USA.

boilermaker's deafness an obsolete term for noise-induced hearing loss, which was particularly prevalent amongst riveters who worked inside boilers and hence encountered very high levels of noise for long periods of time.

bone-anchored hearing aid a hearing aid with a bone-conduction output via a transducer whose vibrating element is directly attached to the cranial bones. *See also* BONE VIBRATOR, BONE-CONDUCTION HEARING AID.

bone conduction the transmission of sound to the inner ear primarily by means of mechanical vibration of the cranial bones (ISO 8253-1). Sound waves from a suitably placed external vibrator, usually behind the ear on the mastoid process, travel through the bones of the skull into the fluid of the cochlea, producing a sensation of hearing.

bone-conduction hearing aid a hearing aid whose output is from a bone-conduction vibrator worn on a headband or in a spectacle arm.

bone-conduction oscillator an obsolete term for a bone vibrator.

bone-conduction transducer *see* BONE VIBRATOR.

bone-conduction receiver *see* BONE VIBRATOR.

bone-conduction vibrator *see* BONE VIBRATOR.

bone conductor *see* BONE VIBRATOR.

bone vibrator an electromechanical transducer intended to produce the sensation of hearing by vibrating the cranial bones (ISO 8253-1). A bone vibrator designed to be used with a hearing aid – fitted when an ear insert is contra-indicated – is normally placed on the mastoid process. Bone vibrators for audiometry may be placed on the mastoid or on the forehead, and are designed to have a circular contact surface of standardized area. Also known as a bone-conduction receiver, bone-conduction transducer, bone-conduction vibrator or bone conductor. *See also* BONE-ANCHORED HEARING AID, BONE-CONDUCTION HEARING AID.

boundary microphone a microphone which is designed to work with a flat plate behind it to give a noise-reducing effect.

brainstem that part of the brain that is on the top of the spinal column, consisting of the medulla oblongata, the pons and the mid-brain. Electrical activity of the brainstem can be detected in response to an acoustic signal at the ear. *See also* AUDITORY BRAINSTEM RESPONSE.

breakthrough at a point in an electronic circuit, the presence of an unwanted signal which originates from the (wanted) signal at another point in the circuit or system. Also known as crosstalk.

brief tone a sinusoidal signal having a duration of less than 200 ms. (IEC 60645-3). Brief tones are mainly used in auditory-evoked-response audiometry. Sometimes called a tone pip. *See* Figure 6 a, under PEAK-TO-PEAK EQUIVALENT SOUND PRESSURE LEVEL *and also* SHORT-DURATION SIGNAL, TONE BURST.

broadband or **broad-band** a term used to describe, for example, a signal or the frequency response of an amplifier, indicating an absence of filtering to constrain the bandwidth. The term wideband is also used.

button cell a flat, circular cell used in hearing aids and other miniature devices, often called a battery.

byte a group of bits, often eight, which specify a character, number or similar information in a digital memory.

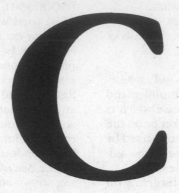

C-weighting a standardized frequency response (i.e., standardized frequency weighting) used mainly in sound level meters for noise measurements. It gives a substantially flat frequency response over the audio-frequency range, in contrast to the A and B weightings which have a reduced response at low frequency. *See* Figure 4, under FREQUENCY WEIGHTING.

CAT *see* COMPUTER-AIDED TRANSCRIPTION.

CEN European Committee for Standardization.

CENELEC European Committee for Electrotechnical Standardization.

CCIR Comité Consultatif International du Radio. A body which issues international recommendations for radio communications and performance standards for radio systems; part of the International Telecommunications Union (ITU).

CCITT Comité Consultatif International du Télégraphique et Téléphonique, the international committee which adopts recommendations for standardization of telecommunications networks and services as well as operational and tariff procedures used throughout the world. It also draws up general plans for international telecommunication networks. Part of the International Telecommunications Union (ITU); now called ITU-T.

CDT *see* CONNECTED-DISCOURSE TRACKING.

CERA *see* CORTICAL-EVOKED-RESPONSE AUDIOMETRY.

CF *see* CHARACTERISTIC FREQUENCY.

CIC aid completely-in-the-canal aid. *See* CANAL AID.

CIS *see* CONTINUOUS INTERLEAVED SAMPLING.

CM *see* COCHLEAR MICROPHONIC.

CMR *see* COMODULATION MASKING RELEASE.

CROS contralateral routing of signals. A hearing-aid system designed for a person with one good, often normal, ear and one totally or profoundly deaf ear. A microphone is placed on the deaf ear and the signal from it is taken across the head, often in a spectacle frame, and fed to an amplifier and then through an earpiece into the good ear, which is not blocked with an earmould. The user benefits by hearing sounds falling on the deaf side without the screening effect that the head would otherwise give. A similar system is BICROS, in which microphones are placed on both sides of the head, for use by a person who has an aidable loss on one side and little or no hearing on the other, with the sound fed into the better ear.

cadence (of speech) the rhythm and/or intonation pattern of speech.

calculated loudness level loudness calculated by a specified procedure (IEC 801-29-06). Such procedures, which involve the combination of measurements of sound level in several frequency bands, are given in British Standard 4198 and ISO 532. *See also* EFFECTIVE PERCEIVED NOISE LEVEL, JUDGED PERCEIVED NOISE LEVEL, LOUDNESS LEVEL, PERCEIVED NOISE LEVEL.

calibration all the operations for the purpose of determining the values of the measurement errors and, if necessary, other metrological properties of a measuring instrument. *Note:* The metrological use of the term 'calibration' is often extended to include operations such as adjustments, scale graduation, etc. This use is deprecated. (BS 4727: Part 1: Group 04 modified).

calibrator *see* SOUND CALIBRATOR.

caloric test a test of the vestibular function of an ear, i.e., which relates to the sense of balance. It involves irrigation of the ear canal with cold and then warm water. This causes convection currents in the fluids in the vestibular labyrinth, resulting in changes in the natural movements of the eye, that can be observed by the tester. *See also* NYSTAGMUS.

canal aid a hearing aid which is small enough to be worn almost entirely within the ear canal; a small version of an in-the-ear aid (ITE aid). Also known as an in-the-canal aid (ITC aid). A completely-in-the-canal-aid (CIC aid) is one that is worn entirely in the ear canal close to the eardrum. *See also* DEEP-CANAL AID.

cans a slang expression for headphones, used by disc jockeys and others.

capacitor microphone *see* CONDENSER MICROPHONE.

capacity of a battery, the amount of charge that the battery can hold, usually expressed as the product of a current and the time for which that current can be supplied, in ampere hours (Ah) or milliampere hours (mAh).

carbon microphone a microphone which depends for its operation on variations in contact resistance between carbon granules (IEC 801-26-12). The granules are disturbed by movement of the microphone diaphragm in response to sound pressure.

cardioid microphone a microphone with a heart-shaped polar response, i.e., most sensitive to a sound source in front of the microphone, with the sensitivity falling as the sound source moves to either side, and greatly reduced for sounds coming from the rear.

Carhart notch a phenomenon by which ears with otosclerosis show, superimposed on the general trend, a dip in the bone-conduction audiogram of typically 15 dB, centred at around 2000 Hz.

carrier frequency the frequency of a carrier signal, i.e., a signal which is used to carry a lower-frequency modulating signal. In radio transmissions the receiver is tuned to the carrier frequency and the carrier signal may be modulated by speech, music or data in a variety of ways. *See also* AMPLITUDE MODULATION, FREQUENCY MODULATION.

carrier phrase a short phrase that precedes the presentation of a test word in speech audiometry, serving to present the test word in a more natural context and to inform the subject that a test word is imminent.

categorical perception a perception process by which a continuously variable set of items are grouped into defined categories, for example the perception of phonemes.

cavitation the production of bubbles in a liquid subject to negative pressure. The violent collapse of such bubbles in response to a rise in pressure produces an intense source of noise, known as cavitation noise.

cent a logarithmic unit of frequency, i.e., a unit of frequency interval. One cent is the interval between two sounds whose fundamental-frequency ratio is the 1200th root of two. An equally-tempered semitone is equal to 100 cents.

central auditory dysfunction a hearing loss which occurs due to a malfunction of the auditory system at a level above the brainstem or in the cortex.

central masking a masking effect which is due to the interaction of signals from both ears at the cortical level.

central processing the processing of a signal at the cortical level.

centre clipping a type of waveform distortion which may be produced by an electronic circuit, usually an amplifier: the input signal is reproduced at the output in a non-linear manner, with low-level sections of the input waveform deleted but high-level sections substantially unchanged. *See* Figure 5, under PEAK CLIPPING.

centre frequency the frequency corresponding to the midpoint of the pass band of a bandpass filter or similar device. Also known as the mid-band frequency.

cerumen ear wax.

characteristic frequency (CF) of a particular cochlear nerve fibre, the frequency to which it most readily responds.

charge amplifier an amplifier designed to accept the signals from a transducer with a very high, essentially capacitative output impedance, for example, from a piezoelectric accelerometer. The use of a conventional amplifier with such a transducer may result in loss of low frequencies and unwanted effects from the capacitance of the input leads.

cholesteatoma a cyst made up of a soft, friable material with a pearly-grey sheen or a yellowish coloration, frequently found in the upper part of the middle-ear cleft. It has invasive properties and can erode ossicles and other organs.

chopped speech speech test material produced by dividing the speech signal into short sections which are fed alternately to each ear. The ability to put the sections together and to understand the speech is an indication of the central speech-processing ability of the listener. *See also* INTERRUPTED SPEECH TEST.

chronic long lasting, i.e., a chronic condition is one of long standing. The opposite of acute.

cilium on a sensory cell of the type found in the cochlea and semi-circular canals, a hair-like process whose movement can trigger a neural output. The plural form of cilium is cilia.

circumaural earphone an earphone having a cavity large enough to cover the region of the head which includes the ear (IEC 801-27-24).

class A, B, C, D a classification of amplifiers according to their mode of operation. In a class-A amplifier, the mean current drain does not vary with the amplitude of the output signal. In a class-B amplifier, the mean current drain rises and falls with the output level, allowing power savings when the output level is low and hence greater overall efficiency. A class-D amplifier operates in a switching mode, i.e., with the output devices rapidly switched between fully 'on' and fully 'off' states, in such a manner that, averaged over the switching cycles, an appropriate current waveform is delivered. The class-D design offers very high efficiency, since very little power is dissipated in the output devices. The class-C design is intended to drive a resonant load and its use is restricted almost entirely to radio transmission. *See also* PUSH-PULL AMPLIFIER.

click a transient acoustic or vibratory signal whose frequency spectrum covers a broad range, often called a broadband click (IEC 60645-3); a short, sharp sound.

clinical audiology that part of audiology which is concerned with the diagnosis of hearing impairment and, often, the rehabilitation of those with hearing loss.

clipping *see* PEAK CLIPPING.

close-talking microphone a specially designed microphone that is placed very close to the lips and is used in noisy situations to ensure a minimum pick-up of background noise relative to the speech signal.

closed-set test an identification test involving a limited number of test items of which the subject has advance notice. For example, subjects may be given a short list of words from which they have to choose the one that they hear. The opposite of an open-set test in which, as far as the subject is aware, there is no restriction on the range of test items.

coaxial cable a cable with a centre conductor surrounded by insulation and then by an outer metal screen, usually of woven metal strands. The term is generally reserved for cables of this type which are designed for use at radio frequencies. *See also* SCREENED LEAD.

cochlea a snailshell-shaped structure, that part of the peripheral auditory system from the oval window to the cochlear nerve, which together with the vestibular system forms the inner ear. *See* Figure 2. under EAR.

cochlear duct the membranous labyrinth of the cochlea, bounded by the basilar membrane and Reissner's membrane, which divides the cross-section of the cochlea in two and which contains the organ of Corti. Also called the cochlear partition or scala media. *See* Figure 2, under EAR.

cochlear echo *see* OTOACOUSTIC EMISSION.

cochlear implant a device based on electrodes implanted in the cochlea which deliver electric currents to excite the auditory nerve and produce a sensation of hearing. The signal for the electrodes is derived from a microphone via a signal processing unit, normally worn on the body. The processed signals from this unit are passed to the electrodes via a transcutaneous transmission system or through a percutaneous plug fitted behind the ear. Used as a hearing aid for profoundly and totally deaf people.

cochlear microphonic (CM) an electrical signal which can be detected by electrodes near or inside the cochlea. The signal follows the pressure waveform of the sound presented to the ear at low and moderate levels, but is limited at high levels.

cochlear nerve *see* AUDITORY NERVE.

cochlear partition *see* COCHLEAR DUCT.

cochleography *see* ELECTROCOCHLEOGRAPHY.

cocktail-party effect the ability of a person in the presence of numerous sounds, incident from sources in various directions, to distinguish one particular acoustical signal, e.g., speech arriving from one particular direction – as might occur when listening to a speaker at a noisy party.

cocktail-party noise noise generated by a large number of people speaking at the same time, as at a cocktail party. Recordings of cocktail-party noise are used as competing signals in hearing tests with speech material. The noise has a long-term spectrum equivalent to that from a typical speaker. *See also* COMPETING SPEECH.

comb filter a filter whose amplitude response, plotted as a function of frequency, shows a regular series of peaks and troughs.

combination tone a tone perceived as a component of a complex stimulus, i.e., a stimulus with two or more frequency components, that cannot be directly associated with any one of the constituent components of the stimulus. For example, when the ear is stimulated with a stimulus having components at f_1 and f_2 (with $f_2 > f_1$), a tone with a pitch corresponding to the frequency ($2f_1 - f_2$) is often heard. In the context of listening to musical notes, the term Tartini tone is sometimes used. *See also* DIFFERENCE TONE, SUMMATION TONE.

comfortable listening level a level at which the listener can listen for an extended period of time, without the sound seeming too loud or too quiet. *See also* MOST COMFORTABLE LISTENING LEVEL.

comodulation masking release the release from masking which may occur when the amplitude-modulation pattern of a masking signal is also present in a similar signal, simultaneously presented in a different frequency region, or when components of a masking signal in different frequency regions have the same pattern of amplitude modulation.

competing speech speech that is used in competition with a speech test signal, i.e., to provide interference or distraction. The competing speech may be continuous, used as a background noise, or its timing may be related to that of the test signals. *See also* COCKTAIL-PARTY NOISE.

completely-in-the-canal aid *see* CANAL AID.

complex signal a signal other than a sinewave.

complex sound a sound other than a pure tone.

compliance *see* ACOUSTIC COMPLIANCE.

comprehensive frequency response a set of frequency responses taken at a number of input levels to show how the performance of an amplifier changes with input level; particularly important for specifying the performance of devices such as hearing aids in which the frequency response changes with input level. *See also* BASIC FREQUENCY RESPONSE.

compressed-speech test a test to determine a subject's ability to comprehend speech which has been compressed in time, i.e., speeded up. This tests for abnormalities of speech processing in the time domain. A decreased ability to process speech is associated with a number of neurological problems, and such effects may be particularly apparent when using time-compressed speech.

compression (1) the reduction in dynamic range of a signal by, for example, an automatic-gain-control system. Also known as output compression (since the dynamic range of the output is reduced compared to that of the input) or amplitude compression. Compression may be used in a hearing aid to accommodate a user with recruitment who can hear comfortably over only a limited range of sound levels. *See also* COMPRESSION RATIO, MULTIBAND COMPRESSION.

compression (2) an increase in local density, and hence in local pressure, corresponding to the positive-going part of an acoustic wavefront. (The negative-going part of a wavefront is associated with a rarefaction, i.e., a reduction in local density and local pressure.)

compression ratio for a system which performs compression of signals, the ratio of the dynamic range of input signals to the dynamic range of output signals. For example, if a 20 dB input range is compressed to a 10 dB output range the compression ratio is 2:1.

compression wave *see* COMPRESSIONAL WAVE.

compressional wave a wave in an elastic medium that causes an element of the medium to change its volume without undergoing rotation (IEC 801-23-04). Sound waves in fluids are examples of a compressional wave: the movement of, for instance, the diaphragm of a loudspeaker causes the air in front of it to be compressed; this compression travels away from the loudspeaker as a compressional wave. Also known as a compression wave or pressure wave.

computer-aided transcription (CAT) transcription of speech by use of electronic processing applied to the input from a skilled operator on a purpose-designed keyboard. Used for transcription in law courts, etc., and to give live transcriptions via a monitor display for use by deaf people. *See also* PALANTYPE, STENOGRAPH, VELOTYPE.

computer-controlled audiometer *see* AUDIOMETER (3).

computer-controlled audiometry measurement of hearing with a computer-controlled audiometer. *See* AUDIOMETER (3).

concha the bowl of the pinna. *See* Figure 2, under EAR.

condensation (in acoustics) in a medium, the fractional change of density which is associated with the presence of a sound wave. (The density is slightly increased from its equilibrium value in regions of positive sound pressure and slightly decreased in regions of negative sound pressure.)

condenser microphone a microphone that operates by variation of electrical capacitance (IEC 801-26-13). Also known as a capacitor microphone or electrostatic microphone. *See also* ELEC-TRET MICROPHONE.

conditioning a process whereby a subject is taught to respond in a certain way to a stimulus. For instance a young child may be taught to put a toy man in a toy boat every time he/she hears a test sound; if the level of the sound is then reduced, an indication of the threshold of hearing can be obtained from noting the point at which the child no longer responds accurately to the test signal. *See also* GO GAME, PLAY AUDIOMETRY, TOY TEST, VISUAL-REINFORCEMENT AUDIOMETRY.

conductive hearing loss a hearing loss due to a blockage in the outer ear, including the ear canal, or a malfunction of the middle ear. In other words, a hearing loss due to a disturbance of any part of the mechanism that conducts sound into the inner ear from the air which surrounds the head. *See also* SEN-SORINEURAL HEARING LOSS.

congenital hearing loss hearing loss due to genetic inheritance. Also known as familial hearing loss, genetic hearing loss or hereditary hearing loss. The term is also used, incorrectly, to indicate any form of hearing loss which is present at, or before, birth.

connected-discourse tracking (CDT) a test procedure to measure the ability of a subject to follow connected speech, phrase by phrase. With information from an audio signal and/or lipreading, the subject has to repeat back the words of a speaker who reads from a text. The task is to achieve 100% accuracy – if necessary by means of repetition, etc., by the speaker. The number of words completed in a given time is the parameter measured. Often called speech tracking. *See also* RUNNING SPEECH.

consonance (1) a recurrence of the same or similar sounds in a word or phrase.

consonance (2) a harmonious, i.e., pleas-

ant sounding, combination of sounds such as musical notes.

consonant a speech sound that is not a vowel.

continuous interleaved sampling (CIS) a signal-coding strategy used in some cochlear implants, whereby the individual electrodes in the cochlea are stimulated sequentially.

continuous spectrum a spectrum, e.g., of a sound, whose components are continuously distributed over a given frequency range (IEC 801-21-17 modified). *See also* LINE SPECTRUM, POWER SPECTRAL DENSITY.

contralateral on the opposite side, i.e., in the hearing context, in the opposite ear.

contralateral masking *see* CONTRALATERAL STIMULATION.

contralateral stimulation a test condition in which one ear receives a test signal and the other ear receives another signal, usually different. Contralateral masking occurs when, with a test signal applied to the ear under investigation, the non-test ear receives a masking signal to prevent the test signal being heard in that ear.

conversational speech speech that is spoken at a natural level and in a conversational manner, containing the variations in delivery that occur naturally; as opposed to much speech test material which is spoken in an idealized manner. Conversational speech may also use the particular vocabulary and syntax appropriate for such a context.

conversion deafness a rarely encountered term used to describe a hearing loss of psychological origin. *See* NON-ORGANIC HEARING LOSS.

cortex the outer layer of the brain. The term is often used to indicate the cerebral cortex, i.e., the surface layer of the cerebrum – the two hemispheres which form the largest division of the brain. *See also* AUDITORY CORTEX.

cortical relating to the cortex.

cortical-evoked-response audiometry (CERA) auditory-evoked-response audiometry for investigation of the response of the cerebral cortex to acoustic stimuli. The cortical evoked response occurs some 50 to 250 ms after the acoustic signal has been presented and indicates that the signal has reached the level of the cortex, even though the listener may not necessarily be aware of it.

counterbalanced a term describing an experimental design in which various conditions or treatments are arranged in different orders across various groups of subjects, in such a way that the effect of a particular condition or treatment cannot be attributed to order.

coupled modes modes of oscillation which are not independent but influenced by the transfer of energy from one mode to another. (IEC 801-24-17). For example, the vibrational modes of the reed in a musical instrument such as the clarinet are coupled to the resonant modes of the pipe.

coupler *see* ACOUSTIC COUPLER, MECHANICAL COUPLER.

crest factor for a signal waveform, the ratio of the peak amplitude to the root-mean-square amplitude, i.e., a measure of the 'peakiness' of a waveform.

critical band a range of frequency, centred at some stated audio frequency, whose width relates to the frequency resolution of the ear at that stated frequency. The critical band may be specified on the basis of several different aspects of auditory perception associated with the frequency domain (for example, loudness of complex sounds, masking from noise bands): the response of listeners to stimuli centred around a particular frequency is found to differ according to whether the stimulus frequency range is wider or narrower than a certain critical range – this critical range being the critical band at that particular frequency. The width of the critical band, i.e., the critical bandwidth, provides an approximate measure of the auditory-filter bandwidth. The critical bandwidth varies with fre-

quency; when measured in hertz, critical bands at higher frequencies are wider than those at lower frequencies. *See also* BARK SCALE, CRITICAL RATIO.

critical damping the minimum damping that will allow a displaced system to return to its initial state without oscillation (IEC 801-24-20). In systems of the mass-on-a-spring type, light damping results in an oscillatory behaviour after a displacement and heavy damping results in a non-oscillatory behaviour. The critical damping condition is at the boundary between these two types of behaviour.

critical period the first few years of life during which the abilities for the perception and production of a first language normally develop. If these skills are not learnt during the critical period it is difficult or impossible to develop normal speech and language subsequently.

critical ratio an approximate measure of the auditory filter bandwidth. For the case when a continuous pure tone is just audible in the presence of a broadband noise, the critical ratio at the tone frequency is calculated as the mean-square acoustic pressure (in Pa^2) of the tone divided by the power spectral density (in $Pa^2\ Hz^{-1}$) of the broadband noise in the region of the tone frequency. The critical ratio is thus equal to the bandwidth within which the broadband noise has a sound pressure level equal to that of the pure tone. The critical ratio is found to be approximately 40% of the auditory critical bandwidth. *See also* CRITICAL BAND.

cross correlation a mathematical procedure to measure similarity in the variations of two quantities, which may be used to compare two signal waveforms.

cross hearing in audiometry, the detection of a signal in the non-test ear due to the presence of a high-level signal in the test ear. This problem can be avoided by applying a suitable masking signal to the non-test ear.

cross masking in audiometry, an effect by which a masking signal in the non-test ear is set too loud, so that it crosses the head and affects the perception of the test signal in the test ear.

crossover frequency for two systems whose peak responses are in different frequency ranges, the frequency at the boundary between the range in which one system responds more strongly and the range in which the other responds more strongly. For example, if a highpass filter and a lowpass filter have a crossover frequency of 500 Hz, then above 500 Hz the highpass filter passes more signal and below 500 Hz the lowpass filter passes more signal; both filters pass signals to the same extent at 500 Hz.

crosstalk *see* BREAKTHROUGH.

crystal microphone a high-impedance microphone in which the active element is a piezoelectric crystal. Crystal elements have nowadays been generally replaced by elements made from ceramic materials.

cue (to speech perception) a source of speech information, e.g., a visual cue, an auditory cue.

cued speech a system used to support the perception of speech by profoundly deaf persons, mainly used in the education of deaf children. The speaker produces hand signs close to the mouth to assist in the discrimination of speech sounds which may be confused when lipreading.

cumulative distribution (of a sound) *see* AMPLITUDE DISTRIBUTION.

current drain the current drawn by an electronic circuit from its power source, usually quoted for battery-operated equipment where it relates to the type and life of the battery. *See also* BATTERY CURRENT.

cushion that part of an earphone, sometimes detachable, which rests against the ear or head. In the case of audiometric earphones the cushion is part of the specification for calibration purposes.

custom-made hearing aid an in-the ear aid which has a case or shell that has been made to fit an individual's ear and whose circuits have been adjusted to suit that individual.

cut-off frequency for a highpass or lowpass filter, the frequency at the boundary between the pass band and the stop band.

cut-off voltage measured across the terminals of a battery, the voltage below which the battery is deemed to be beyond its working range and unsuitable to use. Also known as end-point voltage.

cycle per second an obsolete term for hertz, the unit of frequency.

cylindrical wave a wave of which the wavefronts are coaxial cylinders (IEC 801-23-08). A cylindrical wave is emitted by a line source, i.e., a long, thin source which radiates equally from all points along its length, or by a source with cylindrical symmetry. *See also* PLANE WAVE, SPHERICAL WAVE.

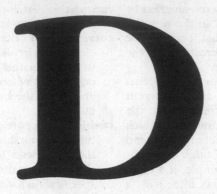

D

d´ pronounced 'dee prime', a measure of the extent to which signals are distinguishable to an observer. For two signals that may be distinguished because of a difference in a certain parameter, e.g., frequency, the value of *d´* is notionally equal to the subjective equivalent of this difference divided by the uncertainty in subjective estimation of the significant parameter. Also known as the index of discriminability or the discrimination index.

dB *see* DECIBEL.

d.c. or **DC** originally serving only as an abbreviation for direct current, the term is now also used in its own right to describe a steady signal or signal component, i.e., a unidirectional constant voltage or current.

DL *see* DIFFERENCE LIMEN.

damping dissipation of the energy of an oscillating system with time or distance. (IEC 801-24-19). *See also* CRITICAL DAMPING, DAMPING RATIO.

damping ratio the ratio of the actual damping to the critical damping. (IEC 801-24-21). In systems of the mass-on-a-spring type, light damping results in an oscillatory behaviour after a displacement and heavy damping results in a non-oscillatory behaviour. The critical damping condition is at the boundary between these two types of behaviour.

dead room a room characterized by a relatively large amount of sound absorption. (IEC 801-31-19). The effect of the absorption is to produce a room which has a short reverberation time, in which a sound undergoes very few reflections before becoming inaudible, giving rise to a 'dead' feel to the room; as opposed to a room which is 'live' and has a long reverberation time, associated with many reflections. An anechoic room is often called a dead room: in fact it represents the limiting case of a dead room, with negligible reflections at the walls within the specified frequency range.

deaf a general term used to describe a person with a hearing loss. However, the term is generally used with a more specific meaning: those who are born profoundly deaf (or who become profoundly deaf before acquiring speech and language), and whose preferred mode of communication is sign language, refer to themselves as deaf. Similarly, those who become profoundly deaf in later life (after acquiring normal speech and language), and prefer to communicate by speech and using lip reading, refer to themselves as deafened; those with a less severe hearing loss who communicate using speech and hearing, often with the help of a hearing aid, refer to themselves as hard of hearing. *See also* HARD OF HEARING, POSTLINGUALLY DEAF PERSON, PRELINGUALLY DEAF PERSON.

deaf aid a commonly used misnomer for a hearing aid.

deaf and dumb a much deprecated term, used incorrectly to describe a person who is deaf and does not have normal speech. A deaf person's inability to produce normal speech is due to an inability to hear and hence establish which sounds are appropriate to produce, not necessarily due to any problems with the speech-production mechanism.

deaf-blind a term used to describe a person who is both deaf and blind. Strictly speaking, the implication is that the person was born deaf and then became blind, or became deaf before becoming blind – a person who was blind and then became deaf would be known as blind-deaf; however, the term deaf-blind is used in practice to cover both cases.

deaf community a term used to describe the cultural grouping of deaf people, generally those who use sign language as their preferred mode of communication.

deaf mute a much deprecated term used incorrectly to describe a person who is deaf and does not have normal speech. A deaf person's inability to produce normal speech is due to an inability to hear and hence establish which sounds are appropriate to produce, not necessarily due to any problems with the speech-production mechanism.

deafened (1) made deaf by illness, noise or accident.

deafened (2) a term used to describe an individual who has become profoundly deaf after acquiring normal speech and language, usually in later life. *See also* DEAF, POSTLINGUALLY DEAF PERSON.

decade (in frequency) a logarithmic unit of frequency, i.e., a unit of frequency interval, corresponding to an increase in frequency by a factor of ten. For example, 10 Hz to 100 Hz is one decade, 63 Hz to 6300 Hz is two decades, etc.

decay rate at a given frequency, the rate at which sound pressure level decreases with time, for example in a room with significant reverberation. (IEC 801-31-08 modified). The unit of decay rate is the decibel per second (dB s^{-1}).

decay time the characteristic time duration associated with a process in which some quantity decreases systematically with time, tending towards a final value (generally a final value of zero). *See also* REVERBERATION TIME, RISE TIME.

decibel (dB) one tenth of a bel. The decibel is the most commonly used unit in acoustics for the measurement of amplitude, power or intensity. A linear scale in decibels corresponds to a logarithmic amplitude scale, thereby compressing a wide range of amplitude values into a small range of numbers. The level difference, in decibels, between two signals of amplitudes a_1 and a_2 is $20\log_{10}(a_1/a_2)$. Similarly the level in decibels of a signal of amplitude a with respect to a reference amplitude a_{ref} is $20\log_{10}(a/a_{ref})$. If the signals are specified in terms of their power W or intensity I, the formulae are similar but the multiplier is 10 rather than 20, i.e., $10\log_{10}(I/I_{ref})$, etc.

Note (1). Letters may be added after the symbol dB to indicate the reference used, as follows:

dB HL (decibels hearing level), i.e., the level of a sound with reference to the standardized average normal threshold of hearing for that sound and for a given method of presentation.

dB HTL (decibels hearing threshold level), i.e., the level of a sound at threshold for a given ear, with reference to the standardized average normal threshold of hearing for that sound and for a given method of presentation.

dB SL (decibels sensation level), i.e., the level of a sound with reference to the threshold of hearing of the particular listener for that sound and method of presentation.

dB SPL (decibels sound pressure level), i.e., the level of a sound with reference to a sound pressure of 20 μPa, the reference pressure used in acoustics.

Note (2). Letters in parentheses following the symbol dB, as in dB(A), dB(B) and dB(C), are used to indicate frequency-weighted sound pressure level, i.e., measured using one or other of the frequency weightings on a sound level meter, with reference to a sound pressure of 20 μPa. Similarly, a flat frequency response may be indicated by dB(Lin). (Although very widely used, this annotation of the dB symbol to indicate frequency weighting is, it may be argued, erroneous because it is the signal that is frequency weighted, not the unit.) *See also* FREQUENCY WEIGHTING.

decibels per decade the unit of slope, i.e., gradient, on a graph of frequency response or spectrum, when the ordinate is plotted in decibels and the abscissa in decades. Used, for example, to describe the fall-off in response of a filter beyond the pass band.

decibels per octave the unit of slope, i.e., gradient, on a graph of frequency response or spectrum, when the ordinate is plotted in decibels and the abscissa in octaves. Used, for example, to describe the fall-off in response of a filter beyond the pass band.

dedicated used exclusively for one task. For example, 'a dedicated microprocessor'.

deep canal aid a hearing aid which is designed to be worn far down the ear canal. *See also* CANAL AID.

delayed auditory feedback a test procedure in which the voice of a subject is fed back to him/her through earphones with a delay in time. After a delay of some 100 ms a normally hearing subject finds difficulty in continuing to speak and may raise the voice, stutter or stop speaking altogether. The test is used to determine non-organic hearing loss. Also called delayed speech feedback or the delayed speech test.

delayed speech *see* DELAYED AUDITORY FEEDBACK.

depth of modulation of an amplitude modulated signal, the maximum fractional change in amplitude produced by the modulation process.

detection (in acoustics) the determination of the presence of a signal (IEC 801-29-34).

detection differential for a specified listener and test procedure, the amount by which the signal level exceeds the noise level presented to the ear for a stated probability of detection. (IEC 801-29-35). For example, the signal-to-noise level corresponding to 50% signal detection.

detection threshold the value of a specified parameter, usually signal level, at which detection of a signal is just possible. The measurement usually involves a specific criterion for detection in a set number of presentations of the test signal. In pure-tone audiometry this is taken to be 50% detection over a stated number of presentations of the pure tone. *See also* DISCRIMINATION THRESHOLD, SPEECH DETECTION THRESHOLD LEVEL, THRESHOLD OF HEARING.

diagnostic audiometry audiometry undertaken with a view to determining the site of a lesion and/or the possible cause of a hearing loss.

diaphragm (in electroacoustics) the sound-reception element of a microphone or the sound-production element of an earphone, generally in the form of a thin, circular sheet which is supported at its edge and attached at its centre to an electromechanical transducer system.

dichotic listening a situation where different stimuli are presented to each ear of a listener. *See also* DIOTIC LISTENING.

difference limen (DL) for a specified parameter of a specified signal, the minimum change in that parameter which can be detected by a subject as a change in that signal. For example, difference limen for frequency, difference limen for intensity. Also known as just noticeable difference (JND).

difference tone an additional tone present at the output of a non-linear system when two tones are applied to the input, whose frequency is equal to the difference between the two input frequencies. For example, inputs at 1000 Hz and 1100 Hz can produce a difference tone at 100 Hz. *See also* COMBINATION TONE, SUMMATION TONE.

differential amplifier an amplifier whose output signal corresponds to the amplified difference between the signals at its two inputs, i.e., an amplifier with a differential input.

differential input an input circuit having two sets of input terminals, the effective input signal being the difference between the electrical signals applied to them.

diffraction (in acoustics) a phenomenon by which a sound wave is changed in direction by an obstacle or other heterogeneity in the medium. (IEC 801-23-25). *See also* REFRACTION.

diffuse field *see* DIFFUSE SOUND FIELD.

diffuse sound field a sound field which in a given region has statistically uniform energy density, and for which the directions of propagation at any point are randomly distributed (IEC 801-23-31). Often simply referred to as a diffuse field. *See also* RANDOM-INCIDENCE SOUND FIELD.

digital device a device, for example, a microprocessor, which operates with digitally coded signals, i.e. binary information, coded as transitions between two discrete states representing the binary digits 0 and 1. *See also* ANALOGUE DEVICE.

digital display a display with a direct indication by means of figures which change to show the appropriate number, as opposed to an analogue display, which indicates via a moving pointer on a scale or dial.

diotic listening a situation where identical stimuli are presented to each ear of a listener. *See also* DICHOTIC LISTENING.

diphthong a vowel which may be perceived as a time-varying sound, such as *oy* in 'boy'.

diplacusis a perceptual disorder in which identical sounds presented to each ear appear to have different tonal characteristics (binaural diplacusis) or in which a single tone presented to one ear is perceived as two tones (monaural diplacusis).

directional gain of a transducer, in decibels, ten times the logarithm to the base ten of the directivity factor (IEC 801-25-68). In other words, the directivity factor expressed in decibels. Also known as directivity index.

directional hearing *see* AUDITORY LOCALIZATION.

directional microphone a microphone whose response is dependent on the direction of sound incidence. (IEC 801-26-06 modified). *See also* OMNIDIRECTIONAL, UNIDIRECTIONAL MICROPHONE.

directional pattern a description, usually presented graphically in polar co-ordinates, of the sensitivity level of an electroacoustic transducer as a function of the direction of propagation of the radiated or incident sound, in a specified plane at a specified frequency (IEC 801-25-66).

directivity factor (1) of an electroacoustic transducer for sound radiation, at a specified frequency, the ratio of the square of the free-field sound pressure at a fixed point on the principal axis to the mean-square sound pressure on the surface of a sphere concentric with the effective acoustic centre of the transducer, and passing through the fixed point (IEC 801-25-67). In other words, a measure of sound radiation in the forward direction in comparison to an average over all directions. *See also* DIRECTIONAL GAIN.

directivity factor (2) of an electroacoustic transducer for sound reception, at a specified frequency, the ratio of the square of the free-field sensitivity to sound waves that arrive along the principal axis to the mean square sensitivity to a succession of sound waves that arrive at the transducer with equal probability from all directions (IEC 801-25-67). In other words, a measure of sound reception in the forward direction in comparison to an average over all directions. *See also* DIRECTIONAL GAIN.

directivity index *see* DIRECTIONAL GAIN.

disability in the context of health experience, a disability is any restriction or lack (resulting from an impairment) of ability to perform an activity in the manner or within the range considered normal for a human being (WHO 1980).

discomfort level (of a sound) *see* LOUDNESS DISCOMFORT LEVEL.

discomfort threshold (for a sound) *see* LOUDNESS DISCOMFORT LEVEL.

discrete frequency component a signal component which is individually distinct in frequency. A sound composed of discrete frequency components will not, therefore, have a continuous spectrum, rather it will have a line spectrum.

discriminability *see d´.*

discrimination in relation to hearing, the ability to determine that one sound is different from another.

discrimination index *see d´.*

discrimination score for a given test subject, a specified test signal and a specified manner of signal presentation, the percentage of correctly recognized test items. When the test items are speech signals this is called the speech recognition score (ISO 8253-3). *See also* DISCRIMINATION THRESHOLD.

discrimination threshold where a subject's discrimination performance depends on a test variable such as signal level, the value for the test variable at which the subject can just discriminate between test signals, corresponding to a given criterion such as 50% correct discrimination. *See also* DETECTION THRESHOLD, DISCRIMINATION SCORE, SPEECH RECOGNITION THRESHOLD LEVEL.

dispersion in an acoustic medium, a change in the speed of sound with frequency.

dissipation of a sound wave, the conversion of sound energy into heat. (IEC 801-31-29). *See also* SOUND ATTENUATION.

dissipation factor the ratio of sound energy dissipated as heat to the energy of the incident sound wave (IEC 801-31-30).

dissonance an inharmonious, i.e., harsh-sounding, combination of sounds.

dissonant harsh sounding, inharmonious.

distortion an undesired change of waveform. Distortion may result from a nonlinear relation between the input and the output of a system or from non-uniform transmission at different frequencies. *See also* HARMONIC DISTORTION, INTERMODULATION DISTORTION, NON-LINEAR DISTORTION

distraction test a hearing test used to screen infants for hearing loss. The child sits on the lap of an adult, generally the mother. One tester, in front of the child, holds the child's attention and a second tester makes a very quiet sound to one side of the child. At 7 months of age a child with normal hearing will give some indication to the tester in front that it has heard the sound. This may be a turn of the head in the direction of the sound or just a slight movement of the eyes in that direction. The sounds may be produced electronically by a hand-held warble-tone generator or by using everyday objects, e.g., rustling tissue paper or running a spoon around the inside of a cup; a high-frequency rattle produced for this purpose by Manchester University may also be used.

Doerfler-Stewart test a test designed to detect the presence of non-organic hearing loss. The test is based on noise interfering with the understanding of speech. Speech and noise levels to the same ear are varied, making it difficult for the listener with non-organic hearing loss to follow accurately and in keeping with the normal effects of such changes in signal-to-noise ratio.

Doppler shift when a fast-moving sound source approaches a listener, or a listener moves rapidly towards a sound source, the consequent increase in the pitch of the sound, as compared to the corresponding no-movement situation. Similarly, the decrease in pitch when the source moves away from the listener or the listener moves away from the source.

double-blind test procedure in a test involving the comparison of two or more test conditions, a procedure by which neither the test subject nor the experimenter performing the test is aware of which test condition is being used.

drift a slow, continuous change in the mean level of a signal or the offset error of an electronic device.

duty cycle of a signal or device which cycles between 'on' and 'off' states, the proportion of time for which the 'on' state is present, normally expressed as a percentage.

dynamic characteristics characteristics which are obtained under other than steady-state test conditions.

dynamic range (1) of a system or device, the range (usually the range of signal intensity) over which normal operation is possible. This range is generally expressed in decibels. In the case of hearing, the dynamic range may be taken from the threshold of hearing to either the loudness discomfort level or the threshold of pain.

dynamic range (2) of a signal parameter,

the range (maximum to minimum) within which that parameter falls. This range is generally expressed in decibels.

dyne an obsolete unit of force. The force required to accelerate a one-gram mass to a velocity of one centimetre per second during one second. Now replaced by the newton: one dyne is equal to 10^{-5} newtons.

dysacousia *see* DYSACUSIS.

dysacusia *see* DYSACUSIS.

dysacusis a perceptual disorder in which the listener reports distortion in hearing. Also called dysacousia or dysacusia.

dysarthrias a group of disorders arising from a range of neurological conditions that adversely affect the production of speech.

dysfunction an abnormality or impairment of function.

dysgraphia an acquired disorder caused by a trauma to the brain which affects the ability to write.

dyslexia difficulty with reading, writing and spelling.

dysphasia difficulty in speaking due to a neurological impairment.

dysphonia a disorder of respiration or vocal-cord function which impairs speech production.

dysprosody inappropriate production of speech in terms of suprasegmental features such as intonation, stress, speaking rate, etc.

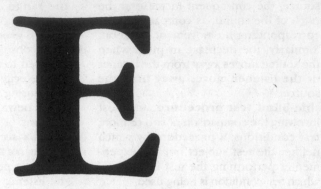

ECoG or **ECochG** *see* ELECTROCOCHLEO-GRAPHY.

EMC electromagnetic compatibility. The EMC evaluation of a piece of equipment involves measurement of its immunity to radiated electromagnetic interference and of the degree to which the equipment itself radiates such interference. *See also* INPUT-RELATED INTERFERENCE LEVEL, OVERALL INPUT-RELATED INTERFERENCE LEVEL.

ENT ear, nose and throat. *See also* OTORHINOLARYNGOLOGIST.

ENT department a hospital department specialising in ear, nose and throat diseases.

ERA evoked-response audiometry *or* electric-response audiometry. *See* AUDITORY-EVOKED-RESPONSE AUDIOMETRY.

ERB *see* EQUIVALENT RECTANGULAR BANDWIDTH.

ETSI European Telecommunications Standards Institute

ear the organ of hearing. The term is often used to refer only to the pinna, which is the external part of the ear. The ear also includes the organs of balance. *See* Figure 2.

ear canal a tubular passage which runs from the pinna to the eardrum. Also called the (external) auditory meatus and the (external) acoustic meatus. *See* Figure 2.

ear defender *see* HEARING PROTECTOR.

ear insert a plug shaped to fit the ear canal, through which the acoustic output from an earphone is delivered. *See also* EARMOULD.

ear light a device used for illuminating the ear canal, for example, when checking the position of tamps placed in the canal to limit the passage of ear-impression material. *See also* OTOSCOPE.

ear pip a term used to describe a small, ready-formed plastic ear insert, often used as a temporary measure until an individually fitted earmould is available. Ear pips also fitted to some types of earphones used with 'Walkman'-type cassette players and radios.

earplug a plug that fits firmly into the ear canal in order to exclude sound or water.

ear protector *see* HEARING PROTECTOR.

ear simulator an alternative term for an artificial ear, but now also used as a generic term for both acoustic coupler and artificial ear.

ear trumpet a purely acoustic hearing aid shaped like a trumpet, with the wider end receiving sound and the narrow end held in the entrance to the ear canal. This provides a limited amount of amplification. Mainly used nowadays by frail elderly people, who favour its simplicity.

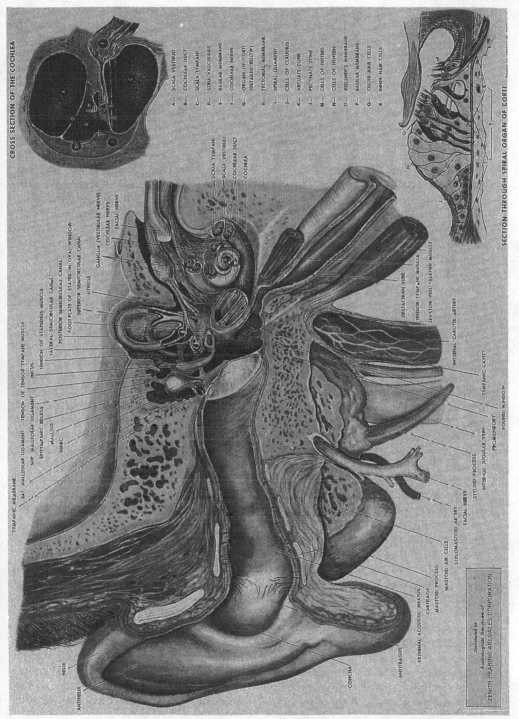

Figure 2. Anatomy of the ear. The diagram indicates the position of organs and structures referred to in the dictionary as well as additional organs and structures that are not referred to. (Reproduced by permission of Zenith Electronics Corporation, Gelnville, Illinois, USA).

Note: AUDITORY NERVE, EAR CANAL and EARDRUM are labelled here by the alternative terms COCHLEAR NERVE, EXTERNAL ACOUSTIC MEATUS and TYMPANIC MEMBRANE, respectively.

eardrum the membrane that closes the inner end of the ear canal and moves in response to sound waves. The anatomical term for the eardrum is the tympanic membrane. *See* Figure 2, under EAR.

earmould a plug shaped to fit an individual ear, made from an impression of that ear, through which the acoustic output from a hearing aid is conveyed to the eardrum. According to the acoustic needs of the wearer, an earmould may completely seal the ear canal, may only partially block the ear canal (in the case of a vented earmould) or may leave the ear canal effectively unobstructed (in the case of an open earmould, as used with the CROS hearing-aid configuration). The earmould should be seen as an integral part of the hearing-aid system as – according to its acoustic design – it can greatly affect the performance of the hearing aid, for better or for worse. *See also* EAR INSERT.

earmuff a hearing protector covering the region of the head which includes the ear. The term is also used for a protective cover over the ear to keep out the cold.

earphone an electroacoustic transducer by which acoustic signals are obtained from electrical signals, and intended to be closely coupled acoustically to the ear (IEC 801-27-18). Earphones are made to fit into the ear canal (*see* INSERT EARPHONE), to be worn against the pinna (*see* SUPRA-AURAL EARPHONE) or to fit around the pinna (*see* CIRCUMAURAL EARPHONE). *See also* HEADPHONE, RECEIVER.

earpiece a general term for a device, or a part of a device, designed to deliver sound to the ear and intended for use near, on or in the ear.

echo a sound wave that has been reflected and arrives with such a magnitude and time interval after the direct sound as to be distinguishable as a repetition of it (IEC 801-31-21). *See also* MULTIPLE ECHO.

effective masking level for a masking noise band, the hearing level to which the threshold of hearing of a notional normal person, for a pure tone whose frequency coincides with the centre of the noise band, is raised by the presence of the noise band.

effective perceived noise level a measure, calculated from sound pressure levels in one-third octave bands, of the noise from a single aircraft overflight as heard on the ground. Used exclusively for the purpose of noise certification as specified by the International Civil Aviation Organization (ICAO). The term is broadly analogous to sound exposure level but there are various differences in the calculation procedure. *See also* CALCULATED LOUDNESS LEVEL, LOUDNESS LEVEL, NOISE EXPOSURE LEVEL, PERCEIVED NOISE LEVEL, SOUND EXPOSURE LEVEL.

efferent nerve a nerve which conveys signals outwards, for example, from the brain to the peripheral organs.

eighth cranial nerve *see* AUDITORY NERVE.

electret microphone a condenser microphone in which the electrostatic field results from an internal permanent charge in one of the capacitor electrodes (IEC 801-26-14 modified). Electret microphones are widely used because they offer good performance at low cost and can be made very small. A pre-amplifier circuit is often incorporated with stand-alone electret microphones.

electric-response audiometry (ERA) *see* AUDITORY-EVOKED-RESPONSE AUDIOMETRY.

electroacoustic transducer a transducer designed to receive an electrical input signal and to furnish an acoustic output signal or vice versa (IEC 801-25-47). *See also* ELECTROMECHANICAL TRANSDUCER.

electroacoustical characteristics the characteristics of a device or system which relate to its electrical and acoustical properties, in particular to the transfer between electrical and acoustic signals, or vice versa.

electroacoustics the subject covering all applications which involve the use of electrical or electronic means to generate, amplify or measure acoustic signals.

electrocochleography (ECochG, ECoG) a method for measuring the electrical potentials within the cochlea that are produced by acoustic stimuli. The measurement uses an electrode on the end of a long needle which is passed through the eardrum to rest on the bony outer wall of the cochlea. *See also* AUDITORY-EVOKED-RESPONSE AUDIOMETRY.

electrode a conducting element via which electrical signals may be introduced into a medium or detected within a medium. *See also* ACTIVE ELECTRODE, INDIFFERENT ELECTRODE.

electrodermal audiometry the measurement of the response to acoustic stimuli by means of changes in skin resistance. *See also* GALVANIC SKIN RESPONSE.

electrodynamic loudspeaker *see* MOVING-COIL LOUDSPEAKER.

electrodynamic microphone *see* MOVING-CONDUCTOR MICROPHONE.

electroencephalograph a device for measuring, via surface electrodes, the electrical signals present on the scalp. These signals may include components which are produced in response to acoustic or other test signals.

electromagnetic loudspeaker a loudspeaker that operates by variation of the reluctance of a magnetic circuit (IEC 801-27-05). Also known as a variable-reluctance loudspeaker.

electromagnetic microphone a microphone that operates by variation of the reluctance of a magnetic circuit (IEC 801-26-16). Also known as a variable-reluctance microphone.

electromechanical transducer a transducer designed to receive an electrical input signal and to furnish a mechanical output signal or vice versa (IEC 801-25-32). *See also* ELECTROACOUSTIC TRANSDUCER.

electronystagmography the measurement of electrical signals, deriving from reorientation of the corneo-retinal potential associated with eye movement. *See also* NYSTAGMUS.

electrophonic effect the production of an auditory sensation by electrical stimulation of the cochlea, the auditory nerve or the auditory cortex (IEC 891-02-59).

electrostatic actuator a device comprising an auxiliary electrode that permits the application of an electrostatic force to the metallic or metallized diaphragm of a microphone in order to obtain a calibration (IEC 801-28-10).

electrostatic loudspeaker a loudspeaker that operates by electrostatic forces (IEC 801-27-03); i.e., the force which moves the sound-producing diaphragm is generated by electrostatic attraction or repulsion.

electrostatic microphone *see* CONDENSER MICROPHONE.

electrotactile aid *see* ELECTROTACTILE EFFECT.

electrotactile effect the production of a touch sensation by electrical stimulation of nerves from the touch receptors in the skin (IEC 891-02-62) modified. In an electrotactile aid, speech-derived electrotactile stimuli are used to transmit limited speech information to the user. *See also* TACTILE SENSATION, VIBROTACTILE EFFECT.

end organ a sensory receptor: the part of a sensory mechanism which is furthest from the brain. The end organ in the auditory system is the cochlea.

end-point voltage *see* CUT-OFF VOLTAGE.

endemic continuously present within a particular community.

endocochlear potential *see* ENDOLYMPH.

endolymph the fluid that fills the cochlear duct. It has high potassium level and low sodium level and an electric potential of + 80 mV with respect to the scala tympani. This potential is known as the endocochlear potential.

endolymphatic hydrops *see* MENIERE'S DISEASE.

envelope *see* AMPLITUDE ENVELOPE.

equal-loudness contour *see* EQUAL-LOUDNESS-LEVEL CONTOUR.

equal-loudness curve *see* EQUAL-LOUDNESS-LEVEL CONTOUR.

equal-loudness-level contour a curve of

sound pressure level versus frequency, connecting points the co-ordinates of which represent pure tones or narrow bands of noise judged equally loud. (ISO 226). Also known as an equal-loudness contour or equal-loudness curve.

equal-loudness-level function for a pure tone of a given frequency or for a narrow band of noise of a given frequency band, the relation between loudness level, expressed in phons, and sound pressure level, expressed in decibels (ISO 226).

equally tempered scale a musical scale formed by division of the octave into 12 equal intervals (IEC 801-30-17). Each of these intervals is an (equally tempered) semitone. In conventional Western music, the equally tempered scale is the standard tuning for fixed-pitch instruments such as the piano. *See also* JUST SCALE, PYTHAGOREAN SCALE.

equally tempered semitone *see* SEMITONE.

equilibrium density of an acoustic medium, the density in the absence of sound. When a sound wave is present, this is associated with small fluctuations in density about the equilibrium value.

equilibrium pressure in an acoustic medium, the pressure in the absence of sound. When a sound wave is present, this is associated with small fluctuations in pressure about the equilibrium value. Also known as static pressure.

equivalent continuous sound level *see* EQUIVALENT CONTINUOUS SOUND PRESSURE LEVEL.

equivalent continuous sound pressure level the root-mean-square sound pressure over a time interval, expressed in decibels (using the standard reference pressure of 20 μPa). Also called time-average sound pressure level. When the measurement is made with a standard frequency weighting, the corresponding quantity is known as equivalent continuous sound level (with the weighting indicated in the title, e.g., A-weighted

equivalent continuous sound level), also known as time-average sound level. The symbol is L_{eq}, sometimes with additions to the subscript, e.g., L_{peq} to indicate equivalent continuous sound pressure level, L_{Aeq} to indicate A-weighted equivalent continuous sound level.

equivalent rectangular bandwidth (ERB) a parameter which specifies the bandwidth of a bandpass filter. The ERB is the area under the curve of power transfer versus frequency for the filter, divided by the value of power transfer at the frequency of peak response.

equivalent threshold sound pressure level (for monaural earphone listening) for a given ear, at a specified frequency, for a specified model of earphone and for a stated force of application of the earphone to the human ear, the sound pressure level set up by the earphone in a specified ear simulator (acoustic coupler or artificial ear) when the earphone is actuated by that voltage which, with the earphone applied to the ear concerned, would correspond to the threshold of hearing (ISO 389).

equivalent volume the volume of an air-filled hard-walled cavity whose acoustic impedance has the same magnitude as that of a given acoustic system. The acoustic impedance of the external ear canal, with the tympanic membrane and its attached structures, is often expressed in terms of an equivalent volume. *See also* TYMPANOMETRY.

etiology *see* AETIOLOGY.

etymotic gain *see* INSERTION GAIN.

Eustachian tube the tube that runs from the nasal cavity into the middle-ear cavity. *See* Figure 2, under EAR.

evoked potential an electrical potential that may be recorded from some part of the brain in response to an external stimulus, e.g., an auditory evoked potential is in response to an acoustic signal at the ear. Also known as an evoked response. *See also* AUDITORY EVOKED RESPONSE.

evoked response *see* AUDITORY EVOKED RESPONSE, EVOKED POTENTIAL.

evoked-response audiometry (ERA) *see* AUDITORY-EVOKED-RESPONSE AUDIOMETRY.

excitation pattern over the set of auditory filters, the distribution of signal with filter centre frequency. The excitation pattern changes with time in response to the time-varying acoustic input.

explosive sound a sound generated by a sudden change in pressure from the equilibrium pressure to a much higher one. *See also* IMPLOSIVE SOUND.

external acoustic meatus *see* EAR CANAL.

external auditory meatus *see* EAR CANAL.

external ear *see* PINNA.

extrapolation when a series of measurements has been taken, for example, at different frequencies, the process of determining values outside the measured range, based on the nature of the set of measured values. *See also* INTERPOLATION.

eyeglass aid *see* SPECTACLE AID.

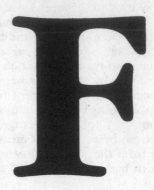

F

F the symbol used to indicate one of the standard time weightings, 'Fast', used in sound level meters. *See* TIME WEIGHTING.

FFT *see* FAST FOURIER TRANSFORM.

FM *see* FREQUENCY MODULATION.

facial nerve the largest nerve running through the middle ear. It leads from the brainstem and controls the facial muscles and virtually all aspects of facial movement. Also known as the seventh cranial nerve or VIIth nerve. *See* Figure 2, under EAR.

falling-ball calibrator a device for checking the calibration of sound-level-meter microphones, which produces a broadband noise at a known sound pressure level due to the action of a large number of small metal balls falling from one side of a compartment to another. Now replaced by sound calibrators, which are electromechanical devices. *See also* SOUND CALIBRATOR.

familial hearing loss *see* CONGENITAL HEARING LOSS.

far field *see* FAR SOUND FIELD.

far sound field the sound field distant from a sound source, where instantaneous sound pressure and particle velocity are substantially in phase (IEC 801-23-30). Often simply referred to as the far field. *See also* NEAR SOUND FIELD.

fast Fourier transform (FFT) a digital signal-processing algorithm used to calculate the spectrum of a signal. *See also* FOURIER ANALYSIS.

feedback the application, to the input of a system, of a signal derived from the output of the system. Feedback may be positive or negative, according to the phase of the signal that is returned to the input. Negative feedback reduces the gain of a system, and is commonly used to set the gain in amplifier circuitry. Positive feedback may lead to instability in a device, leading to uncontrolled oscillation (e.g., the whistle that is often heard from a hearing aid with a badly fitting earmould, in which sound from the output is picked up by the microphone). *See also* ACOUSTIC FEEDBACK.

fenestra ovalis *see* OVAL WINDOW.

fenestra rotunda *see* ROUND WINDOW.

fenestration a surgical operation performed in the 1940s to overcome the problems of otosclerosis. Now replaced by the stapedectomy operation.

filter a frequency-selective system. *See also* ACTIVE FILTER, BANDPASS FILTER, HIGHPASS FILTER, LOWPASS FILTER, NOTCH FILTER.

filtered click a sound generated electronically by bandpass filtering a pulse signal. *See also* SHORT-DURATION SIGNAL.

finger spelling or fingerspelling a system of using the fingers to indicate letters. In the UK two hands are used to indicate the letters whereas in the USA only one hand is used. *See* Figure 3.

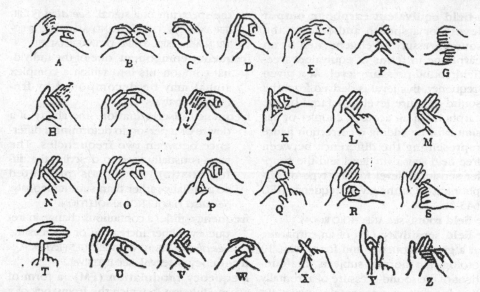

Figure 3. Finger spelling. The two-handed manual alphabet as used in the UK.

foetal audiometry audiometry undertaken on the foetus by means of sounds presented through the stomach wall. The fact that the sound has been heard is indicated by measuring physiological changes such as heart rate.

forced-choice test a test where the subject has to make a choice between two or more test stimuli. In a hearing test the listener has to make a choice between two or more acoustic signals, for example: 'Which of these three sounds is the odd one out?'.

forced oscillation an oscillation maintained by a periodic external excitation (IEC 801-24-01).

formant one of a number of local maxima in the spectrum of a vowel sound, corresponding to resonances in the vocal tract of the speaker. The frequency at each maximum is a formant frequency – these are numbered $F1$, $F2$, etc., starting with the lowest frequency. Vowels are distinguished primarily by differences in formant frequencies, produced by changes in shape of the speaker's vocal tract.

formant frequency *see* FORMANT.

formant transition a rapid change in formant frequency that occurs at the beginning of a vowel sound following a consonant. Formant transitions, particularly the second-formant transition, provide an acoustic cue to the preceding consonant.

forward masking a phenomenon whereby the detectability of a signal is reduced in the period just following a masking noise. Also known as post-stimulatory masking. *See also* BACKWARD MASKING.

Fourier analysis the decomposition of a signal waveform, or a mathematically described function, into a set of sinusoidal components. The amplitudes, frequencies and phases of these components provide a full specification of the original waveform or function. After a theorem stated by Joseph Fourier, who lived in France at the time of Napoleon. The mathematical procedure for Fourier analysis is known as the Fourier transform. *See also* FAST FOURIER TRANSFORM.

Fourier transform *see* FAST FOURIER TRANSFORM, FOURIER ANALYSIS.

free field *see* FREE SOUND FIELD.

free-field equivalent earphone output level for a speech audiometer, the sound-pressure level generated by an earphone in terms of equivalent free-field sound-pressure level. At a given frequency, this level is derived from the sound-pressure level generated by the earphone in an acoustic coupler or ear simulator by adding a correction figure representing the difference between free field sensitivity level and the coupler sensitivity level for the type of earphone used at the given frequency (IEC 645-2).

free-field room *see* ANECHOIC ROOM.

free-field sensitivity (1) of an earphone, at a given frequency and for at least 10 otologically normal subjects, the quotient of the sound-pressure of a frontally incident plane progressive wave (0° sound incidence) and of that voltage of equal frequency which is applied to the terminals of the earphone in order that the subjects, on average, judge the sound wave and the sound produced by the earphone as equally loud; both sounds being received in the same ear (IEC 645-2).

free-field sensitivity (2) of an electroacoustic transducer for sound reception, for a specified frequency and a specified direction of sound incidence, the quotient V/p of the open-circuit voltage V and the sound pressure p in the undisturbed plane-progressive free field (IEC 801-25-54 modified).

free progressive wave a wave propagating in a medium, free from boundary effects (IEC 801-23-03).

free sound field a sound field whose boundaries exert a negligible effect on the sound waves. Often simply referred to as a free field. *See also* QUASI-FREE FIELD.

frequency the rate at which a periodic phenomenon occurs, i.e., the number of cycles per second. The unit of measurement is the hertz (Hz).

frequency analysis a general term describing procedures for determining the spectrum of a signal. *See also* FOURIER ANALYSIS, OCTAVE-BAND ANALYSIS, SPECTRUM ANALYSER, THIRD-OCTAVE ANALYSIS.

frequency component one of the individual components into which a complex signal may be decomposed by frequency analysis.

frequency discrimination the ability of a device or a person to determine a difference between two frequencies. The term is usually used to describe the differentiation of signals presented sequentially rather than simultaneously. *See also* FREQUENCY RESOLUTION.

frequency glide a continuous change in frequency, either increasing or decreasing. *See also* GLIDE TONE, SWEEP GENERATOR.

frequency interval *see* INTERVAL.

frequency modulation (FM) a form of modulation in which the frequency of a carrier signal is varied (either side of its mean frequency) according to a modulating signal. For example, the frequency of a nominal 1 MHz carrier might vary from 999 kHz to 1001 kHz in response to small troughs and peaks in the modulating signal, and from 990 kHz to 1010 kHz in response to larger-amplitude features.

frequency resolution the ability of a device or a person to distinguish between different frequency components which are simultaneously present in a signal. Good frequency resolution allows separation of a frequency-specific signal from background noise. Also known as frequency selectivity. *See also* FREQUENCY DISCRIMINATION.

frequency response of a device, the amplitude response (i.e., the ratio of the output amplitude to the input amplitude), plotted as a function of frequency. In acoustics a frequency response is usually plotted on a logarithmic frequency scale, with the amplitude response a_{out}/a_{in} plotted in decibels as $20\log_{10}(a_{out}/a_{in})$. *See also* PHASE RESPONSE, TRANSFER FUNCTION.

frequency selectivity *see* FREQUENCY RESOLUTION.

frequency sweep *see* SWEEP GENERATOR.

frequency transposition the moving of a signal from its original frequency range to a lower, or higher, range. Used in some hearing aids with the intention of bringing high-frequency consonants into a lower frequency range where the wearer has residual hearing.

frequency weighting (1) in a sound level meter, filtering which may be applied to the signal which is being measured.

frequency weighting (2) a descriptor indicating the frequency response of the filtering circuitry in a sound level meter, standardized as 'A' , 'B' or 'C' in IEC 651 which is currently under revision. The 'B' weighting is now deemed obsolete. An absence of frequency weighting, i.e., a flat or linear frequency response, is indicated by Lin. *See* Figure 4. *See also* A-WEIGHTING, B-WEIGHTING, C-WEIGHTING, DECIBEL.

fricative a high-frequency speech sound produced by forcing the airstream through a narrowed aperture in the vocal tract, e.g., *s* in 'see'. For an unvoiced fricative such as *s*, the vocal cords do not vibrate; for a voiced fricative such as *z*, vocal-cord vibration (i.e., phonation) contributes an additional component to the sound. *See also* MANNER OF ARTICULATION.

full-on acoustic gain the air-to-air gain of a hearing aid when the volume control is turned to its maximum position.

functional hearing loss *see* NON-ORGANIC HEARING LOSS.

fundamental frequency for a periodic signal, the frequency corresponding to the repetition rate. The spectrum of a periodic signal with fundamental frequency f will, in general, contain components at f, $2f$, $3f$, etc., although one or more of these components may be absent (including, sometimes, the component at the fundamental frequency f). *See also* MISSING FUNDAMENTAL.

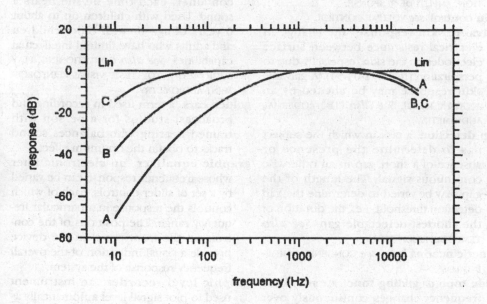

Figure 4. Frequency weighting curves for sound level meters.

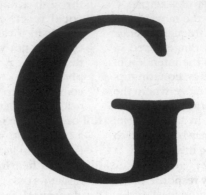

gain for an amplifying system, the ratio of the output amplitude to the input amplitude. For most audio systems the gain G is commonly expressed in decibels, as $20\log_{10}G$, this being equivalent to the difference between the level of the output signal and the level at the input. *See also* AIR-TO-AIR GAIN, AMPLIFICATION, AMPLITUDE RESPONSE.

gain control *see* VOLUME CONTROL.

galvanic skin response the change in electrical resistance between surface electrodes on the skin, especially due to perspiration (IEC 891-04-54). A galvanic skin response may be elicited by an acoustic signal. *See also* ELECTRODERMAL AUDIOMETRY.

gap detection a task in which the subject has to determine the presence or absence of a short gap in an otherwise continuous signal. The length of the gap may be varied to determine the gap detection threshold, i.e., the duration of the shortest detectable gap. *See also* TEMPORAL RESOLUTION.

genetic hearing loss *see* CONGENITAL HEARING LOSS.

glide tone *or* **gliding tone** a tone whose frequency changes continuously over time, either increasing or decreasing. *See also* FREQUENCY GLIDE.

glue ear a condition which causes the middle ear to be filled with a thick glue-like fluid. The medical term is chronic otitis media with effusion.

go game a means of obtaining a response to auditory signals from very young children. The child is taught to place a brick in a box, or some other object into a container, each time he/she hears a sound. Used with children up to about 6 years of age or with older children and adults who have limited intellectual capabilities. *See also* CONDITIONING, PLAY AUDIOMETRY, TOY TEST, VISUAL-REINFORCEMENT AUDIOMETRY.

golden ears a term used in recording and broadcast studios for a person with trained hearing who balances sound tracks to obtain the optimum effect.

graphic equalizer an electronic filter whose frequency response can be varied by a set of slider controls, each of which controls the response in a particular frequency range. The positions of the controls on the front panel of the device provide a visual indication of the overall frequency response of the system.

graphic level recorder an instrument used to plot signal level automatically as a function of time. Also known simply as a level recorder.

grommet a small tube which, with minor surgery, may be inserted into the eardrum so as to ventilate the middle ear when a secretory middle-ear condition such as glue ear is present.

gun microphone a microphone with a long extension which gives the appearance of a rifle or long-barrel pistol. The extension forms an acoustic array that gives the microphone a high degree of directionality. *See also* LINE MICROPHONE.

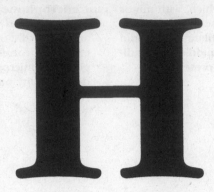

HAIC Hearing Aid Industry Conference. An organization in the USA which produced some of the first methods for specifying hearing aid performance and continues to work in this area.

HATS *see* HEAD AND TORSO SIMULATOR.

HL *see* DECIBEL, HEARING LEVEL.

HTL *see* DECIBEL, HEARING THRESHOLD LEVEL.

Hz *see* HERTZ.

Haas effect for two brief sounds in close succession which are heard as a single sound, e.g., an impulse and its echo, the effect by which the apparent location of the overall source is determined largely by the source location of the first sound, even if the later sound is as much as 10 dB more intense. Also known as the precedence effect. A similar phenomenon may be observed in the case of signals such as speech: if the voice of a talker is enhanced by a public-address system, the talker may be perceived as the sole sound source providing the amplified sound is suitably delayed.

habituation a reduction in response to a constant signal resulting from central processing. *See also* ADAPTATION, AUDITORY FATIGUE.

hair cells cells that lie along the basilar membrane in the cochlea and respond to acoustic stimulation. *See* Figure 2, under EAR. There are three rows of outer hair cells and a single row of inner hair cells. It is now generally accepted that the sensory response of the inner hair cells is enhanced by vibrations generated in the outer hair cells in response to the acoustic input.

half-peak elevation in a speech audiogram, the difference in decibels between the half peak level of the individual subject and the half-peak level of the reference speech recognition curve. *See also* REFERENCE SPEECH RECOGNITION CURVE.

half-peak level *see* half-optimum speech level.

half-optimum speech level in speech audiometry, for a given test subject, for a specified speech signal and a specified manner of signal presentation, the speech level at which half of the maximum speech recognition score is obtained and which is lower than the optimum speech level(s) (ISO 8253-1). Used when there is no level at which the subject can achieve a 100% score and in particular where the maximum score is less than 50%. *See also* HALF-PEAK ELEVATION.

handicap a disadvantage for a given individual, resulting from an impairment or a disability, that limits or prevents the fulfilment of a role that is normal (depending on age, sex and social and cultural factors) for that individual. (WHO 1980). In the case of hearing the impairment is the loss of hearing, the disability is the fact that the person cannot hear speech and other sounds as normal, and the handicap will depend upon the activity that the person undertakes. The handicap is therefore situation specific.

hard of hearing a term which describes an individual whose hearing loss is such that he/she may benefit from using a hearing aid. The International Federation of the Hard of Hearing (IFHOH) states that the expression 'hard of hearing' means: all people who have a hearing loss and whose usual means of communication is by speech. It includes those who have become totally deaf after the acquisition of speech. *See also* DEAF, DEAFENED.

harmonic (1) in a periodic signal (other than a sinewave), a frequency component at a frequency which is an integral multiple of the fundamental frequency. A harmonic can be labelled to indicate its relation to the fundamental frequency, for example, in a signal with a fundamental frequency of 120 Hz, a component at 600 Hz is the fifth harmonic. *See also* HARMONIC SERIES, OVERTONE, PARTIAL.

harmonic (2) of a frequency, an integral multiple of that frequency. A harmonic can be labelled to indicate its relation to the underlying frequency; for example, 600 Hz is the fifth harmonic of 120 Hz. *See also* HARMONIC SERIES, SUBHARMONIC.

harmonic distortion distortion which produces harmonics. In other words, distortion such that a sinusoidal signal becomes non-sinusoidal and hence its spectrum acquires harmonic components. Such distortion occurs when a sinewave passes through a non-linear system. For a device such as an amplifier, with a sinewave input, harmonic distortion can be characterized in terms of the total harmonic distortion (THD): the root-mean-square amplitude of the harmonic components in the output signal, as a percentage of the amplitude

of the output component at the input frequency. A THD of 0.01%, for example, indicates very-high-quality reproduction and a figure of 10% indicates poor quality. *See also* INTERMODULATION DISTORTION.

harmonic series a set of values, usually a set of frequencies, in the ratio 1:2:3:4 etc. For example, 125 Hz, 250 Hz, 375 Hz, 500 Hz, 625 Hz, etc. *See also* OVERTONE, PARTIAL.

harmonic series of sounds a series of sounds within which the fundamental frequency of each sound is an integral multiple of the lowest fundamental frequency (IEC 801-30-04 modified).

head and torso simulator (HATS) a device which simulates the principal acoustic properties of the average adult head and torso, e.g., the effect of the head on the sound field at the ear. Such a device is described in IEC Technical Report 959. Also known as artificial head and torso, artificial manikin or KEMAR (Knowles Electronic Manikin for Acoustical Research) when describing one manufacturer's particular version.

head shadow when sound is incident from one side of the head, the effect by which the sound level at the opposite ear is reduced compared to that at the ear which faces the source.

headband aid a hearing aid in which the greater part of the aid is housed in a case mounted on a band which fits over the head. Sound may be conducted into the ear by means of an acoustic tube, a lead with an external earphone or one with a bone vibrator. *See also* SPECTACLE AID.

headphone or **headphones** an assembly of one or two earphones on a headband (IEC 801-27-20).

headroom in an amplifier, the maximum amount by which the signal can be increased from the nominal working level without distortion due to abnormal operation. *See also* OVERLOAD INDICATOR.

headset an assembly of a microphone and one or two earphones on a headband (IEC 801-27-21).

hearing the subjective perception of sound.

hearing aid a wearable instrument intended to aid a person with impaired hearing, usually consisting of a microphone, amplifier and earphone or bone vibrator, powered by a low-voltage battery (IEC 801-28-20). *See also* MASTER HEARING AID.

hearing conservation measures to prevent hearing loss. For example, the use of hearing protectors in a noisy working environment.

hearing disability a disability brought about by the inability to perceive everyday sounds, this inability resulting from a hearing impairment.

hearing handicap a handicap arising from a hearing disability.

hearing handicap index a measure of the overall hearing capability of a person, obtained using a self-assessment questionnaire: the person is asked to judge his/her ability to hear a variety sounds under various conditions.

hearing-impaired person one who has a hearing impairment.

hearing impairment a physical or psychological malfunction of the auditory system. *See also* IMPAIRMENT.

hearing instrument an alternative term for a hearing aid.

hearing level (HL) for a specified signal, for a specified type of transducer and for a specified manner of application, the sound pressure level (or the vibratory force level) produced by the transducer in a specified acoustic coupler or artificial ear (or mechanical coupler) minus the appropriate reference equivalent threshold sound pressure level (or reference equivalent force level) (IEC 645-1). In practice, in pure-tone audiometry, this means the level of a test signal with respect to audiometric zero and therefore the value indicated on the hearing-level dial.. *See also* DECIBEL, HEARING LEVEL FOR SPEECH, HEARING THRESHOLD LEVEL.

hearing level for speech for a specified speech signal and a specified manner of signal presentation, the speech level minus the appropriate reference speech recognition threshold level (ISO 8253-3). In practice, in speech audiometry, this means the level of the test material with respect to the specified reference level for that test material. Also known as speech hearing level. *See also* SPEECH LEVEL.

hearing loss the effect of a hearing impairment, i.e., a loss of hearing sensitivity and/or discrimination ability. Usually described in terms of the cause of the loss and the degree of loss as demonstrated on a pure-tone or speech audiogram. *See also* HEARING THRESHOLD LEVEL.

hearing protector a device placed within the ear canal, in the concha, over the ear, or over a substantial part of the head to protect the ear from noise (IEC 801-28-21). Also called an ear protector or ear defender.

hearing therapist in the UK, a person trained to undertake the rehabilitation of hearing-impaired adults. The term is also used in the USA to describe a peripatetic teacher of the deaf. *See also* SPEECH AND LANGUAGE THERAPIST.

hearing threshold *see* THRESHOLD OF HEARING.

hearing threshold level (HTL) for a specified signal and method of presentation, the amount in decibels by which the threshold of hearing for a listener exceeds a specified standard threshold of hearing (IEC 801-29-24 modified). In practice, in pure-tone audiometry, this means the level of a test signal at threshold, with respect to audiometric zero. *See also* DECIBEL, HEARING LEVEL. The term 'hearing loss' is often used in clinical practice to describe the hearing threshold level of an impaired ear, as indicated on an audiogram.

helicotrema the region at the apex of the cochlea where the scala vestibuli joins the scala tympani. *See* Figure 2, under EAR.

helix a fold in the pinna. *See* Figure 2, under EAR.

Helmholtz resonator an acoustical resonator, i.e., a system which responds to sound only within a narrow frequency range, consisting of a relatively large air-filled cavity linked to the surrounding air via a hole or tube (for example, in the shape of a wine bottle).

hereditary hearing loss *see* CONGENITAL HEARING LOSS.

hertz the SI unit of frequency, symbol Hz. *See also* FREQUENCY.

heterodyne a term used to describe the technique in which two sinewaves of different frequencies are simultaneously applied to a non-linear device in order to produce an output component at a frequency equal to the difference of the two input frequencies. The principle is used, for instance, in radio receivers to reduce the frequency of the received signal to a lower, fixed frequency that can be more easily handled. *See also* BEAT-FREQUENCY OSCILLATOR.

hi-fi *see* HIGH FIDELITY.

high fidelity related to an audio amplifier system, the term indicates high-quality reproduction in which the output signal is very nearly identical in form to the input signal. Often abbreviated to hi-fi.

high-frequency audiometry pure-tone audiometry in the frequency range 8 kHz to 16 kHz, using equipment described in IEC 60645-4.

high-frequency boost a relative increase in high frequencies due to the action of some part of an amplifying system. In hearing aids the user-control position to achieve such an effect is marked with an *H. See also* BASS BOOST, BASS CUT, HIGH-FREQUENCY CUT.

high-frequency cut a relative decrease in high frequencies due to the action of some part of an amplifying system. In hearing aids the user-control position to achieve such an effect is marked with an *L* to indicate low-frequency emphasis (which is equivalent to high-frequency cut). *See also* BASS BOOST, BASS CUT, HIGH-FREQUENCY BOOST.

high-tone loss a hearing loss affecting perception of sound at higher frequencies, above 1kHz, say.

highpass filter or **high-pass filter** a filter, specified by a particular cut-off frequency, which attenuates signals at frequencies below the cut-off. Signals at frequencies above the cut-off are allowed to pass with negligible attenuation. *See also* LOWPASS FILTER.

homophasic of the same phase.

homophone a word pronounced in the same way as another but having a different spelling and meaning. For example, *horse* and *hoarse* are homophones.

horn *see* ACOUSTIC HORN.

horn loudspeaker a loudspeaker in which the radiating element is coupled to the medium by means of a horn (IEC 801-27-13).

howl around *see* ACOUSTIC FEEDBACK.

howl back *see* ACOUSTIC FEEDBACK.

hum (1) in mains-operated equipment, or in other electronic equipment operated in the vicinity of mains wiring, the unwanted mains frequency or its harmonics that are present at the output of the device.

hum (2) a low-pitched continuous sound.

hummers a term used to describe people who can detect continuous very-low-frequency noise in the environment when others cannot.

hydrodynamic noise when an object moves through a fluid, or fluid flows past an object, sound which may be radiated as a result of local pressure fluctuations induced by unsteady flow. When the fluid is air, the term aerodynamic noise may be used.

hydrophone a transducer that produces electrical signals in response to water-borne acoustic signals (IEC 801-32-26).

hyperacusis abnormal acuity of hearing.

hypoacusis hearing loss.

hysteric hearing loss hearing loss of a non-organic origin, often brought on by some sudden trauma. *See also* NON-ORGANIC HEARING LOSS.

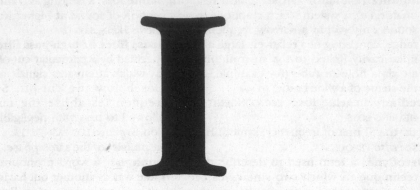

I the symbol used to indicate one of the standard time weightings, Impulse, used in sound level meters. *See* TIME WEIGHTING. Also the symbol for electrical current.

IEC International Electrotechnical Commission.

IPA *see* INTERNATIONAL PHONETIC ALPHABET.

ISO International Organization for Standardization.

ITC aid in-the-canal aid. *See* CANAL AID.

ITE aid *see* IN-THE-EAR AID.

ITU, ITU-T International Telecommunications Union. See CCIR, CCITT.

iatrogenic a term used to describe an ill effect caused by the implementation of a medical examination or treatment.

idiopathic a term used to describe a disease of unknown cause.

immittance a general term denoting either impedance or admittance (IEC 801-25-16). *See also* ACOUSTIC IMMITTANCE.

immittance audiometry *see* TYMPANOMETRY.

impact noise a noise due to the mechanical excitation of a structure by the impact of driving force, for example, the sound created by footfalls on a floor or banging on a partition.

impaired hearing *see* HEARING IMPAIRMENT.

impairment loss or abnormality of psychological, physiological or anatomical function leading to a disability and possible handicap.

impedance a characteristic quantity describing the behaviour of a medium or system in respect of waves or signals, defined in terms of a complex quotient. For example, electrical impedance is voltage divided by the corresponding current. *See also* ACOUSTIC IMPEDANCE.

impedance matching the procedure by which maximum power transfer between two parts of an acoustic system, or electrical circuit, is achieved by matching the acoustic impedance, or electrical impedance, at the interface between the two parts.

implant *see* COCHLEAR IMPLANT, MIDDLE-EAR IMPLANT.

implosive sound a sound generated by a sudden change in pressure from the equilibrium pressure to a much lower one. *See also* EXPLOSIVE SOUND.

impulse noise noise consisting of an irregular sequence of impulsive sounds.

impulsive sound a sound, such as a gunshot, which occurs for a short period of time.

in-situ gain (of a hearing aid) the gain of a hearing aid when measured on a standardized artificial head and torso, thus corresponding to the gain that would be achieved on an average human head. Also known as simulated in-situ gain.

See also AIR-TO-AIR GAIN, INSERTION GAIN.

in-the-canal aid (ITC aid) *see* CANAL AID.

in-the-ear aid (ITE aid) a hearing aid worn entirely within the outer ear. Also known as an intra-aural aid. *See also* CANAL AID.

inaudible sound a sound that cannot be heard because it is below the threshold of hearing or outside the frequency range of audibility.

incidence the number of cases of a disease occurring, generally within a specified locality and within a specified period.

incus the middle bone in the ossicular chain. *See* Figure 2, under EAR.

index of discriminability *see d´*.

indifferent electrode an electrode which acts as a reference, for example, in a balanced three-electrode system which feeds into a differential amplifier. Also known as a reference electrode. *See also* ACTIVE ELECTRODE.

induction (in electromagnetism) the generation of a voltage in a conductor due to a changing magnetic field in the vicinity of the conductor, or due to the conductor moving within a magnetic field.

induction coil (1) in a hearing aid, a small coil of wire with a large number of turns which is intended to pick up the audio-frequency magnetic field from an induction loop system or a suitably designed telephone. By selecting the *T* switch position on the hearing aid instead of the microphone *M* position, the induction coil is switched into circuit in place of the hearing-aid microphone. Also called an induction pick-up coil or pick-up coil (PUC). *See also* T.

induction coil (2) a coil in a telephone handset, often placed around the earphone, used to generate a magnetic field for use with hearing aids in the same manner as an induction loop.

induction loop for hearing aid users, a system which produces an audio frequency magnetic field which can be picked up by an induction coil in the hearing aid when this is switched to the 'T' position. The magnetic field is generated by the current in a wire loop driven from an amplifier with an input from a microphone, tape recorder, etc. The main advantage of the 'loop' system is that it minimizes the effects of distance and background noise for the hearing-aid user.

induction pick-up coil *see* INDUCTION COIL (1).

industrial audiometry audiometry that is undertaken as part of a hearing conservation programme in industries that have a noisy working environment.

industrial deafness hearing loss that may be attributed to working in a noisy environment or due to exposure to sudden loud noise in the workplace. Also known as occupational hearing loss.

inertance a quantity representing the inertia of an acoustic system. In a system whose behaviour is dominated by inertia, the inertance at a given surface is equal to the sound pressure divided by the volume acceleration. An inertance M_A contributes a term of magnitude $2\pi f M_A$ to the acoustic impedance at frequency f. Also known as acoustic inertance or acoustic mass.

infinite baffle an extensive plane surface in which a loudspeaker may be mounted to provide an effectively infinite air path between the front and the rear of the loudspeaker diaphragm. In practice this air path must be at least 10 wavelengths at the lowest frequency to be reproduced. *See also* ACOUSTIC BAFFLE.

infrasonic *see* INFRASOUND.

infrasound acoustic oscillation whose frequency is below the low-frequency limit of audible sound (about 16 Hz) (IEC 801-21-03). The adjective is infrasonic (or, rarely, subsonic). *See also* ULTRASOUND.

inherent noise noise that is generated within an electrical circuit or a device and not present as a result of external influences or due to malfunction. In audio amplifying devices this is usually heard as a rushing sound, due to the broadband nature of the signal. Also known as self noise. *See also* SHOT NOISE, THERMAL NOISE.

inner ear that part of the peripheral auditory system from the oval widow to the cochlear nerve, i.e., the cochlea, together with the vestibular system. *See* Figure 2, under EAR.

input/output function a graph showing the relationship, at a specific frequency, between the amplitude of the input signal to an amplifying device and that of the output. In hearing aids this graph indicates departures from a linear response and the effects of limiting and compression at higher levels of output.

input-related interference level (IRIL) a parameter used to characterize the immunity of a hearing aid to electromagnetic interference, in particular that from GSM and other mobile phones using digital transmissions. The IRIL expresses the interference at the output of the hearing aid as an equivalent acoustic input to the microphone. The IRIL is measured in decibels sound pressure level using a 1 kHz test signal. Decreasing values of IRIL indicate increasing immunity. *See also* OVERALL INPUT-RELATED INTERFERENCE LEVEL.

insert earphone a small earphone that fits either in the outer ear or is attached directly to a connecting element, for example an earmould inserted in the ear canal (IEC 801-27-22). A button-type earphone as used with bodyworn hearing aids. Also known as an ear insert.

insertion gain (of a hearing aid) when an external sound source is present, the gain corresponding to the difference between the sound pressure level in the ear canal with and without the hearing aid being present. The term insertion gain is generally reserved for a measurement on an artificial head and torso. For measurement on a person wearing a hearing aid the term real-ear insertion gain is generally used. Also known as etymotic gain. *See also* AIR-TO-AIR GAIN, IN-SITU GAIN.

instantaneous sound pressure *see* SOUND PRESSURE.

integrating-averaging sound level meter an instrument for the measurement of the equivalent continuous sound pressure level L_{eq} and optionally sound exposure level, described in IEC 804 Integrating-Averaging Sound Level Meters. A frequency-weighting network may be used, e.g., for measure A-weighted equivalent continuous sound level L_{Aeq}.

integration time the period of time over which a time average or sum over time is taken. If varying weighting is applied to different parts of the time window, an effective integration time may be quoted – generally less than the overall duration of the time window. *See also* TIME WEIGHTING.

intelligibility (of speech) a general term indicating the extent to which speech is understood by a listener, used to indicate the clarity with which speech is produced or reproduced, as heard by a normal listener, or the extent to which clearly produced speech is understood by a hearing-impaired listener.

intelligibility score in speech audiometry, an obsolete term for what is now known as speech recognition score.

intensity *see* SOUND INTENSITY.

interaural between the ears.

interaural amplitude difference the amplitude difference between sound falling on each ear by virtue of the location of the sound source with respect to the listener's head. Such amplitude differences can be used by the listener to localize the source. *See also* AUDITORY LOCALIZATION, HEAD SHADOW.

interaural attenuation the difference in level which occurs when an acoustic stimulus is applied to one ear of an individual and measured at the other ear, in corresponding position and acoustical conditions.

interaural time difference the time difference between sound falling on each ear by virtue of the location of the sound source with respect to the listener's head. Such time differences can be used by the listener to localize the source. *See also* AUDITORY LOCALIZATION.

interference (1) a phenomenon that results from the superposition of two or more waves of the same frequency but different in phase or direction of propagation (IEC 801-23-13).

interference (2) unintended extraneous signals which may be superimposed on the intended signal. *See also* SPEECH INTERFERENCE LEVEL.

interference patterns patterns of maximum and minimum intensity that arise from the interference of two or more waves.

interferometry a method of measuring interference patterns or making them visible.

intermodulation distortion distortion which occurs when two signals (or, in the general case, more than two) are passed through a non-linear system, producing distortion components at the various sum and difference frequencies between integral multiples of the frequency of the one signal and integral multiples of the frequency of the other signal. Usually measured with pure-tone test signals. *See also* HARMONIC DISTORTION.

internal acoustic meatus *see* INTERNAL AUDITORY MEATUS.

internal auditory meatus the passage through which the auditory nerve runs from the cochlea. *See* Figure 2, under EAR. Also known as the internal acoustic meatus.

internal impedance in an electrical source such as a signal generator or battery, an impedance inherent in the device which is determined by the electrical, physical or chemical construction.

The internal impedance is apparent in terms of the fall in output voltage which occurs when a significant current is drawn. If the internal impedance is a pure resistance, it may be referred to as the internal resistance.

internal resistance *see* INTERNAL IMPEDANCE.

international phonetic alphabet (IPA) an internationally agreed set of letter-like symbols, each representing a phoneme, used for the representation of speech. *See also* PHONETIC SYMBOL.

interpolation when a series of measurements have been taken, for example, at different frequencies, the process of determining intermediate values that have not been measured, based on the nature of the set of measured values. *See also* EXTRAPOLATION.

interrupted speech test a test of speech perception where the speech test material is interrupted in time. *See also* CHOPPED SPEECH.

interval the spacing in frequency between two periodic sounds or signals, e.g., two musical notes, measured in terms of the ratio of their (fundamental) frequencies or, more often, the logarithm of that ratio. Also known as frequency interval or pitch interval. *See also* DECADE, OCTAVE, SEMITONE, TONE.

intonation modulation or rise and fall in the pitch of the voice. The intonation pattern carries suprasegmental speech information. *See also* CADENCE, SUPRASEGMENTAL SPEECH FEATURES.

intra-aural in the ear.

intra-aural aid *see* IN-THE-EAR AID.

ipsilateral on the same side, i.e., in the hearing context, in the same ear.

isophonic a term used to describe sounds which have the same loudness.

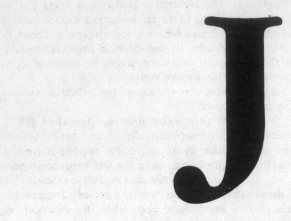

JND or jnd just noticeable difference. *See* DIFFERENCE LIMEN.

jack or jack plug a cable-mounted, electrical signal connector with coaxial contact surfaces and a distinctive waisted tip; designed to push fit into a matching socket. Jack plug/socket combinations can be designed to perform electrical switching operations, for example, to disconnect a loudspeaker when headphones are plugged in.

Johnson noise *see* THERMAL NOISE.

judged perceived noise level the sound pressure level, in decibels, of a frontally presented octave band of pink noise centred on 1 kHz and lasting for two seconds, that is judged equally noisy as a given sound (IEC 801-29-10). *See also* EFFECTIVE PERCEIVED NOISE LEVEL, LOUDNESS LEVEL, PERCEIVED NOISE LEVEL.

just noticeable difference (JND) *see* DIFFERENCE LIMEN.

just scale a musical scale whose frequency intervals are chosen to give major and minor triads with frequencies in the ratio 4:5:6 and 10:12:15 respectively (IEC 801-30-16). *See also* EQUALLY TEMPERED SCALE, PYTHAGOREAN SCALE.

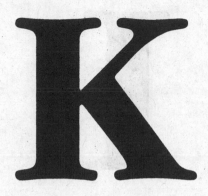

KEMAR Knowles Electronic Manikin for Acoustic Research. A trade name for a widely used version of a standardized head and torso simulator. *See* HEAD AND TORSO SIMULATOR.

kHz *see* KILOHERTZ.

Kemp echo an alternative term for cochlear echo. Named after D T Kemp who discovered the phenomenon. *See* OTOACOUSTIC EMISSION.

kilo the SI prefix denoting one thousand.

The abbreviation is k. For example, 1 kHz (i.e., one kilohertz) is 1000 Hz.

kilocycles per second an obsolete term for kilohertz.

kilohertz a unit of frequency, one thousand hertz. The symbol is kHz. *See also* KILO.

kinaesthesia self-awareness of movement and position. The American spelling is kinesthesia.

kinesthesia *see* kinaesthesia.

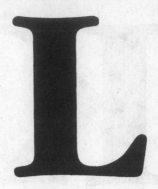

LDL *see* LOUDNESS DISCOMFORT LEVEL.

L_{eq} the symbol for equivalent continuous sound pressure level or equivalent continuous sound level.

labial of the lips. Used, for example, to describe speech sounds whose production involves the lips. *See also* PLACE OF ARTICULATION.

laboratory microphone a high-quality calibrated microphone used for measuring purposes, usually a condenser microphone.

labyrinth the structure of cavities within the temporal bone that contains the inner ear, i.e., the cochlea and the vestibular system.

lapel microphone a microphone for positioning on the clothing of the user (IEC 801-26-26), usually worn on the lapel of a jacket or clipped on a tie. Also known as a tie-clip microphone. *See also* LAVALIERE MICROPHONE.

laryngeal pertaining to the larynx.

laryngology the study of the throat, pharynx, etc., and their function.

laryngograph an instrument for recording laryngeal movements by means of electrodes positioned on the throat.

larynx the part of the windpipe which contains the vocal cords. More colloquially known as the voicebox.

lateralization when sounds are presented through headphones or a bone vibrator, the location by the listener of their apparent position within the head. *See also* AUDITORY LOCALIZATION.

lavaliere microphone or **lavalier microphone** a microphone which is worn as a loop, necklace or lavaliere around the neck. *See also* LAPEL MICROPHONE.

lesion damage to an organ or tissue.

level the logarithm of the ratio of a given quantity to a reference quantity of the same kind. The base of the logarithm, the reference quantity and the kind of level must be indicated. The kind of level is indicated by the use of a compound term such as sound power level or sound pressure level (IEC 801-22 01). Level is a general term used to indicate magnitude when a quantity is measured in logarithmic units. *See also* DECIBEL.

level indicator an indicator on an instrument showing the amplitude or strength of a signal, often scaled in an arbitrary manner.

level recorder *see* GRAPHIC LEVEL RECORDER.

limiter a device to limit the output of a system, used in amplifiers, tape recorders, etc. to prevent overloading the equipment. Used in hearing aids to limit the maximum acoustic output to a level tolerable to the user.

line amplifier an amplifier designed to increase the level of a signal before it is transmitted along a length of cable, The intention is to minimize the effect of interference caused by stray signals picked up on the cable and the effect of losses due to the cable itself.

line microphone a directional microphone, consisting of an array of transducer elements arranged in a straight line, or the acoustic equivalent of such an array. *See also* GUN MICROPHONE.

line spectrum a spectrum, e.g., of a sound, containing only discrete frequency components (IEC 801-21-16 modified). *See also* CONTINUOUS SPECTRUM.

linear a term used to describe a relationship between variables that can be expressed as a straight line in Cartesian co-ordinates. *See also* LINEAR RESPONSE, REGRESSION LINE.

linear response (1) a system response (for example, of an amplifier) which gives an output free from harmonic distortion and intermodulation distortion, specified mathematically in terms of its superposition properties: if input x produces output X and input y produces output Y then input $(x+y)$ produces output $(X+Y)$. *See also* NON-LINEAR RESPONSE.

linear response (2) a flat frequency response over a specified frequency band. On a sound level meter, such a response is indicated by 'Lin'. *See* Figure 4, under FREQUENCY WEIGHTING.

linear system a system with a linear response, in the sense of (1) above.

linearity the relationship between two quantities such that the change in one is exactly and directly proportional to the change in the other.

linguistics the science of language.

lip microphone a microphone designed for use in contact with the lips (IEC 801-26-25), normally used in noisy situations to minimize background noise.

lip reading or **lipreading** the ability to understand a person speaking, with no auditory clues, by observing the lips, face and body language. Also called speech reading or speechreading.

lip-sync the synchronization of recorded speech with a speaker's lips on film or video, when the two have been recorded on different systems.

liquid (consonant) *see* MANNER OF ARTICULATION.

Lissajous figures the figures that result from applying sinusoidal signals to both the X and Y inputs of an oscilloscope. If the two signals have frequencies in integer ratio, a stationary lobed pattern is produced, the details of which relate to the relative frequency, amplitude and phase of the two signals.

listen to give attention to a sound. To listen to a sound is a voluntary action, i.e., a person may choose to listen to a sound but has no control over hearing it.

live room a room characterized by a relatively small amount of sound absorption (IEC 801-31-14). *See also* DEAD ROOM.

live voice a term used in speech audiometry to denote that the tester is using his/her own voice rather than recorded test material.

localization *see* AUDITORY LOCALIZATION.

logarithmic scale a scale on which a variable such as frequency may be represented, such that equal distances along the scale correspond to the same multiplicative factor in the variable. For example, 2, 20, 200 and 2000 Hz are equally spaced on a logarithmic scale of frequency, as are 5, 10, 20 and 40 Hz.

logarithmic unit a unit which applies when a quantity (e.g., amplitude, frequency) is re-expressed in terms of the logarithm of the magnitude of the quantity. For example, the decibel is a logarithmic unit of amplitude, the octave is a logarithmic unit of frequency.

logatom a monosyllabic or polysyllabic speech sound that has no meaning to the listener, often called a nonsense syllable.

Lombard effect the increased loudness of speech which occurs when a speaker is unable to hear his/her own voice because of the presence of loud sound. Particularly noticeable when the interfering sound is presented via headphones.

longitudinal wave a wave in which the direction of particle displacement at each point of the medium is normal to the wavefront (IEC 801-23-05), i.e., parallel to the direction of wave propagation. *See also* TRANSVERSE WAVE.

loop system *see* INDUCTION LOOP.

loudness that attribute of auditory sensation in terms of which sounds may be ordered on a scale from soft to loud (IEC 801-29-03). *See also* LOUDNESS LEVEL, SONE.

loudness-balance the act of adjusting one sound to have equal loudness to another sound, which may be of the same type or of a different type. The two sounds are generally presented alternately, either to the same ear (monaural loudness balance) or to different ears (binaural loudness balance).

loudness balance test *see* ALTERNATE BINAURAL LOUDNESS-BALANCE TEST.

loudness discomfort level (LDL) for a particular type of sound, the level of that sound at and above which a listener experiences discomfort, for reason of excessive loudness. Also known as discomfort level, discomfort threshold, threshold of discomfort, uncomfortable listening level (ULL).

loudness level of a sound, in phons, numerically equal to the median sound pressure level in decibels, *re* 20 μPa, of a free progressive wave having a frequency of 1000 Hz presented to listeners having normal hearing facing the source that in a specified number of trials is judged equally as loud as the unknown sound (IEC 801-29-05). In essence, the loudness level of a sound is numerically equal to the sound pressure level of a 1 kHz tone which is judged to be equally loud. *See also* CALCULATED LOUDNESS LEVEL, JUDGED PERCEIVED NOISE LEVEL, PERCEIVED NOISE LEVEL.

loudness recruitment *see* RECRUITMENT.

loudness scaling the relation between the subjective loudness of sounds and their physical magnitudes.

loudspeaker a transducer by which acoustic waves are obtained from electrical oscillation waves and designed to radiate acoustic power into the surrounding medium (IEC 801-27-01). *See also* MOVING COIL LOUDSPEAKER, ELECTROSTATIC LOUDSPEAKER.

low frequency a relative term to denote a frequency in the lower part of the frequency range under consideration.

low pitch *see* PERIODICITY PITCH.

lowpass filter or **low-pass filter** a filter, specified by a particular cut-off frequency, which attenuates signals at frequencies above the cut-off. Signals at frequencies below the cut-off are allowed to pass with negligible attenuation. *See also* HIGHPASS FILTER.

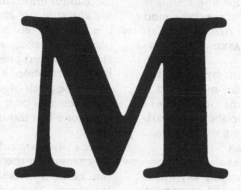

MAF *see* MINIMUM AUDIBLE FIELD.

MCLL *see* MOST COMFORTABLE LISTENING LEVEL.

magnetostriction loudspeaker a loudspeaker that operates by the magnetostrictive deformation of a material (IEC 801-27-07), i.e., the change in dimensions which occurs in a ferromagnetic material when subjected to a magnetic field.

magnetostriction microphone a microphone that operates by the magnetostrictive properties of a material (IEC 801-26-20), i.e., in which distortions of a ferromagnetic material gives rise to an electric current.

magnitude estimation a subjective process in which a numerical value is given by a subject in order to rate some aspect of a test signal.

Makaton a simplified form of sign language which may be used with people who have learning difficulties.

malingering in the context of audiology, the deliberate falsification of responses to audiometric test signals, by the person being tested, in order to exaggerate a hearing loss.

malleus the first bone of the ossicular chain; it is attached to the eardrum at one end and the incus at the other. *See* Figure 2, under EAR.

manikin *see* HEAD AND TORSO SIMULATOR.

manikin unoccluded ear gain the increase in sound pressure produced by the interaction of a manikin with an incident sound field, i.e., the difference between the sound pressure level measured in the ear of the manikin, resulting from a particular incident sound, and the free-field sound pressure level produced by the same sound at the same point in the absence of the manikin.

manner of articulation of a consonant, a classification based on the degree and type of vocal-tract constriction which is involved in the production of the sound. The principal classifications are fricative, stop (plosive), nasal, liquid, semi-vowel and affricate. *See also* PLACE OF ARTICULATION.

manual alphabet *see* FINGER SPELLING.

manual audiometer *see* AUDIOMETER (4).

manual audiometry measurement of hearing with a manual audiometer. *See* AUDIOMETER (4).

masked threshold *see* EFFECTIVE MASKING LEVEL, MASKING.

masker (1) a sound which produces masking. Also known as a masking signal or masking sound.

masker (2) *see* TINNITUS MASKER.

masking (1) the process by which the

threshold of hearing for one sound is raised by the presence of another sound (IEC 801-29-31). *See also* BACKWARD MASKING, FORWARD MASKING, NARROW-BAND MASKING.

masking (2) the amount by which the threshold of hearing for one sound is raised by the presence of another sound, expressed in decibels (IEC 801-29-31). *See also* EFFECTIVE MASKING LEVEL.

masking signal *see* MASKER.

masking sound *see* MASKER.

master hearing aid a hearing aid whose performance can be widely varied. Mainly used for experimental purposes and often not in a wearable form.

mastoid process the protuberance of the skull behind the ear, usually free from hair. *See* Figure 2, under EAR.

maximum acoustic output the maximum sound pressure level that an acoustic transducer or system can deliver to the medium in which it operates. *See also* OSPL$_{90}$.

meatus a channel or passage in the body. *See* EAR CANAL.

mechanical coupler a device designed to present a specified mechanical impedance to a bone vibrator applied with a specific static force, and equipped with a mechano-electric transducer to enable the alternating force level at the surface of contact between vibrator and mechanical coupler to be determined. IEC 60318-6 specifies such a device. *See also* ARTIFICIAL MASTOID.

mechanical impedance (at a point) in a linear mechanical system, the quotient of a force applied at a point, and the resulting component of velocity in the direction of the force. *Note*: In the case of torsional mechanical impedance, the words 'force' and 'velocity' are replaced by 'torque' and 'angular velocity' (IEC 801-25-26). *See also* ACOUSTIC IMPEDANCE.

mechanical reactance the imaginary part of a mechanical impedance (IEC 801-25-28).

mechanical resistance the real part of a mechanical impedance (IEC 801-25-27). *See also* ACOUSTIC RESISTANCE.

mel a unit of pitch. A pure tone frontally presented, having a frequency of 1000 Hz and a sound pressure level of 40 dB, has, by definition, a pitch of 1000 mels. *Note:* The pitch of a sound is judged by the listener to be *n* times that of a 1000 mels tone is *n* thousand mels (IEC 801-29-02).

Ménière's disease a disease characterized by changes to the endolymphatic system in the inner ear and the semicircular canals. The typical symptoms are sensorineural hearing loss, dizziness and/or tinnitus and they may occur at intervals with periods of respite. Also known as endolymphatic hydrops.

method of adjustment a method of measuring subjective response in which the subject is asked to adjust the test signal so as to match a standard signal or achieve a particular condition, for example the detection of a signal at threshold. *See also* PAIRED COMPARISON.

method of constant stimuli a method of measuring subjective response in which the test subject is presented with a number of stimuli, differing in terms of the parameter of interest, and required to indicate in each case whether the stimulus is greater or less than a standard stimulus or whether a particular condition, for example signal detection, has been achieved. *See also* PAIRED COMPARISON.

method of limits a method of measuring subjective response in which the test signal parameter of interest is increased (or decreased) systematically until the subject indicates that a standard signal has been matched or that, for example, signal detection at threshold has been achieved.

micro the SI prefix denoting one millionth. The abbreviation is μ. For example, 1 μPa (i.e., one micropascal) is one millionth of a pascal.

micropascal a unit of pressure, one millionth of a pascal. The symbol is μPa.

The reference sound pressure, corresponding to 0 dB sound pressure level, is 20 μPa for air.

microphone an electroacoustic transducer by which electrical signals are obtained from acoustic oscillations (IEC 801-26-01). *See also* CONDENSER MICROPHONE, ELECTRET MICROPHONE, ELECTRODYNAMIC MICROPHONE, ELECTROMAGNETIC MICROPHONE, PRESSURE-GRADIENT MICROPHONE, PRESSURE MICROPHONE.

microphonic a signal produced by a system whose waveform derives from the system's acoustic environment. For example, an output from a microphone which is not exposed to an airborne sound but is subject to vibration. *See also* COCHLEAR MICROPHONIC.

mid-band frequency *see* CENTRE FREQUENCY.

middle ear that part of the ear from the eardrum to the round window into the cochlea. *See* Figure 2, under EAR.

middle-ear implant a form of hearing aid in which the output signal is a vibration applied directly to the ossicles.

middle-ear reflex *see* ACOUSTIC REFLEX.

mild hearing loss *see* AUDIOMETRIC DESCRIPTOR.

Minicom the commercial name of a particular manufacturer's text telephone.

minimum audible field (MAF) the sound pressure level which relates to the normal binaural threshold of hearing as measured in a free field. ISO 389-7 gives standard values over the audible frequency range. Because the presence of a listener disturbs the sound field, the measurement of sound pressure level is made with the listener absent. *See also* AUDIOMETRIC ZERO, REFERENCE EQUIVALENT THRESHOLD SOUND PRESSURE LEVEL.

missing fundamental a pitch or tone at the fundamental frequency of a complex periodic sound which, in certain circumstances, is heard by the listener even though this frequency is not actually present in the spectrum of the sound. *See also* PERIODICITY PITCH.

mixed hearing loss a hearing loss which

contains both a conductive and a sensorineural element.

mobilization a term used to describe a surgical operation to free the stapes in cases where otosclerosis has restricted its movement.

modal value where the occurrence of the values of some variable may be described by a probability distribution (or, equivalently, by a frequency distribution), the value of the variable which corresponds to the peak of the distribution, i.e., the value which occurs most often. For a continuous variable, e.g. hearing threshold level measured over a number of subjects, the frequency distribution (probability distribution) will be plotted as a histogram, from which the underlying continuous distribution and its modal value may be inferred.

moderate hearing loss *see* AUDIOMETRIC DESCRIPTOR.

modular hearing aid an in-the-ear hearing aid where each model is made to a fixed design and the outer case is not shaped to fit an individual ear. The aid may be used with an ear pip or with an earmould made individually for the user, depending on the model of aid.

modulation the variation of the amplitude or frequency of one, usually continuous, signal so as to follow a second signal. *See also* AMPLITUDE MODULATION, FREQUENCY MODULATION, PULSE-CODE MODULATION.

monaural hearing hearing with one ear.

monaural loudness balance *see* LOUDNESS BALANCE.

mono a prefix, derived from the Greek, meaning single. *See also* MONOPHONIC.

monophasic pulse a pulse, e.g., a current or voltage pulse, in which the signal excursion is in one direction only, either positive or negative. Also known as a monopolar pulse or a unipolar pulse. *See also* BIPHASIC PULSE.

monophonic a term used to describe a sound system with a single channel. Often abbreviated to mono. *See also* QUADRAPHONIC, STEREOPHONIC.

monopolar pulse *see* MONOPHASIC PULSE.

monosyllable a word having only a single syllable. Single words used for measurement of speech recognition are generally chosen as monosyllables, spondees or trochees. *See also* POLYSYLLABIC.

(on a) monotone without a change in pitch.

morpheme the smallest meaningful linguistic segment. The word 'cooks' contains two morphemes, 'cook' and 's', each of which gives linguistic information. *See also* PHONEME, SYLLABLE.

morphology the study of form, particularly the form and structure of living things.

most comfortable listening level or **most comfortable loudness level (MCLL)** the sound pressure level which a person considers to provide the most comfortable loudness for listening to speech or music for a considerable period of time. The MCLL for speech is not necessarily the level which gives maximum speech recognition score. *See also* COMFORTABLE LISTENING LEVEL.

motor theory the theory that, in speech perception, a listener makes reference to information relating to speech production. Now largely discredited.

moving-coil loudspeaker a loudspeaker that operates by the motion of a conductor or coil, carrying a varying current, in a steady magnetic field (IEC 801-27-06). Also called an electrodynamic loudspeaker.

moving-coil microphone a moving-conductor microphone in which the conductor has the form of a coil (IEC 801-26-19).

moving-conductor microphone a microphone that operates by generation of an electromotive force in a conductor moving in a magnetic field (IEC 801-26-17), i.e., the signal voltage is generated by a conductor whose motion in a magnetic field follows that of the sound-receiving diaphragm. Also called an electrodynamic microphone. *See also* MOVING-COIL MICROPHONE, RIBBON MICROPHONE.

multiband compression a speech-processing technique in which bandpass filters are used to split the input speech signal into a number of frequency bands. The signals in each of the bands are individually subject to compression and then combined to give the output signal.

multiple echo a succession of separate echoes originating from a single sound source (IEC 801-31-22).

musical scale a fixed series of sounds, ascending or descending in order of frequency according to a specified scheme of frequency intervals (IEC 801-30-14). *See also* EQUALLY TEMPERED SCALE, JUST SCALE, PYTHAGOREAN SCALE.

myringoplasty a surgical operation to repair perforations in the eardrum by means of grafts.

myringotomy a surgical operation to make an incision in the eardrum.

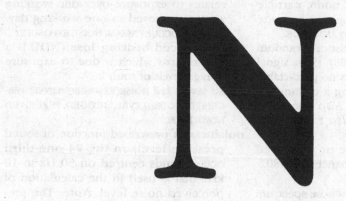

N *see* NEWTON.

NIHL *see* NOISE INDUCED HEARING LOSS.

narrowband or **narrow-band** a term used to describe a noise or a filter, generally taken to imply a bandwidth of 1/2 octave or less.

narrow-band masking in audiometry, the use of one-third-octave or half-octave bands of noise to mask pure tones.

nasal (consonant) a consonant whose production involves the passage of air and sound through the nose. *See also* MANNER OF ARTICULATION.

natural frequency a frequency of free oscillation of a system. For a multiple-degree-of-freedom system, the natural frequencies are the frequencies of the normal modes of oscillation (IEC 801-24-08). For example, the oscillation frequency of a mass on a spring.

near sound field the sound field near a sound source, where instantaneous sound pressure and particle velocity are substantially out of phase (IEC 801-23-29). Often simply referred to as the near field. *See also* FAR SOUND FIELD.

negative feedback *see* FEEDBACK.

neonate a new born child.

neper a rarely used unit of level. One neper is approximately 8.7 decibels.

nerve deafness a term used colloquially to describe sensorineural hearing loss.

neural hearing loss a hearing loss which is caused by a lesion in the auditory neural pathways.

neuro-otology that branch of otology which is concerned with the diagnosis and treatment of hearing and balance problems that are caused by lesions in the neural pathways.

newton a unit of force. The force required to accelerate a one-kilogram mass to a velocity of one metre per second during one second. A force of one newton over an area of one square metre is equivalent to a pressure of one pascal. The symbol is N.

nipple (on an earphone) a term used to describe the raised and shaped central part of a button-type hearing-aid earphone which is the sound outlet and on to which an earmould is clipped. Also called the nub of the earphone.

node a point, line or surface in a standing wave where some specified characteristic of the wave field has essentially zero amplitude. *Notes*: (1) In practice, this amplitude is generally not zero but simply a minimum. The node is then said to be partial. (2) The appropriate modifier should be used before the word 'node' to signify the type that is intended; e.g., displacement node, particle velocity node, sound pressure node (IEC 801-23-16). *See also* ANTINODE.

noise (1) an erratic or statistically random oscillation (IEC 801-21-08), i.e., a signal whose waveform follows no predictable pattern, generally having a continuous broadband spectrum. Also known as random noise. *See also* PINK NOISE, WHITE NOISE.

noise (2) a disagreeable or undesired sound or other disturbance (IEC 801-21-08).

noise band a noise signal whose spectrum is limited to a particular range of frequencies.

noise-cancelling microphone a microphone that discriminates against ambient noise from certain directions or distances (IEC 801-26-11). Also known as an anti-noise microphone.

noise-excluding headset a headset in which each earphone is surrounded by an ear cap, often additional, to provide increased attenuation of ambient noise.

noise exposure a quantity intended to represent the total sound energy received by the ear over a stated time interval. The noise exposure is the time integral, over the interval or event, of the squared instantaneous A-weighted sound pressure. Note that this is essentially the same quantity as sound exposure, except that the integration in this case is normally taken over an eight-hour working day.

noise exposure level noise exposure expressed in decibels, calculated using the formula $10\log_{10}$ (sound exposure/reference exposure). The reference exposure, is usually taken as 11.52×10^{-6} Pa^2 s, corresponding to a pressure of 20 μPa integrated over eight hours. Note that this quantity is closely related to sound exposure level. *See also* EFFECTIVE PERCEIVED NOISE LEVEL, OCCUPATIONAL NOISE EXPOSURE.

noise immission level a similar quantity to noise-exposure level, except that the calculation of noise immission level relates to exposure over one working year, as opposed to one working day. *See also* OCCUPATIONAL NOISE EXPOSURE.

noise induced hearing loss (NIHL) a hearing loss which is due to exposure to high levels of sound.

noise level *see* NOISE EXPOSURE LEVEL, PERCEIVED NOISE LEVEL, JUDGED PERCEIVED NOISE LEVEL.

noisiness a prescribed function of sound pressure levels in the 24 one-third octave bands centred on 50 Hz to 10 kHz that is used in the calculation of perceived noise level. *Note:* The prescribed function is given in ISO 3891 1978 (IEC 801-29-12). *See also* NOY.

nominal value the value given by a manufacturer to a particular performance characteristic.

non-linear distortion distortion that occurs when a signal passes through a system with a non-linear response. *See also* HARMONIC DISTORTION, INTERMODULATION DISTORTION.

non-linear response a system response (for example, of an amplifier) which gives a distorted output. A non-linear response is specified mathematically in terms of failing to satisfy the superposition properties which specify a linear response – in practice, this means that a sinusoidal input signal produces a non-sinusoidal output. A system with a non-linear response will produce harmonic distortion and intermodulation distortion.

non-linear system a system with a non-linear response.

non-organic hearing loss hearing loss which arises due to a psychological reason, i.e., which is not due to an organic problem. Also known as functional hearing loss, psychogenic hearing loss. *See also* HYSTERIC HEARING LOSS, MALINGERING.

non-test ear the ear which is not the subject of the test signal. *See also* TEST EAR.

nonsense speech test material that is not recognizable as meaningful words. *See also* LOGATOM, SYNTHETIC SENTENCES.

normal auditory sensation area the region enclosed by the curves defining the normal threshold of hearing and the normal threshold of pain as functions of frequency (IEC 801-29-28).

normal threshold of hearing *see* REFERENCE EQUIVALENT THRESHOLD SOUND PRESSURE LEVEL.

normal threshold of pain (in electro-acoustics) the modal value of the threshold of pain for a large number of otologically normal listeners between 18 and 30 years of age (IEC 801-29-23).

notch filter a filter which significantly attenuates signals or signal components within a narrow frequency range, while passing signals or signal components at frequencies above or below this range.

note (1) a conventional sign used to indicate graphically the pitch or frequency and duration of a musical sound, and its position in a musical scale (IEC 801-30-06).

note (2) in musical acoustics, a sound sensation or the physical oscillation causing the sensation (IEC 801-30-06).

noy the unit of noisiness, equal to the noisiness of a one-third-octave band of noise centred on 1 kHz and having a sound pressure level of 40 dB. (IEC 801-29-13).

nub (of an earphone) *see* NIPPLE (ON AN EARPHONE).

nystagmus an involuntary rhythmic movement of the eyes. It may be induced by a variety of stimuli designed to aid the diagnosis of vestibular dysfunction, through the interaction of neural activity of the eyes and the organs of balance. *See also* ELECTRONYSTAGMOGRAPHY.

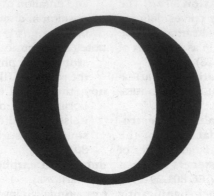

OAE *see* otoacoustic emission.

OIML International Organization of Legal Metrology.

OIRIL *see* OVERALL INPUT-RELATED INTERFERENCE LEVEL.

OSPL$_{90}$ the output sound pressure level from a hearing aid for an input sound pressure level of 90 dB at a specified frequency (or frequencies). The method of measurement is specified in IEC 118-0. *See also* SATURATION SOUND PRESSURE LEVEL.

objective audiometry measurement of hearing in which the person being assessed is not required to make an active response to the test signal. The response is measured in terms of a physiological or electrophysiological effect, e.g., a change in the acoustic impedance at the eardrum (tympanometry) or electrical activity in the auditory neural system (auditory-evoked-response audiometry).

objective tinnitus *see* TINNITUS.

occluded ear an ear in which the ear canal is blocked (occluded) at its outer end, for example, by an earphone.

occluded-ear simulator an acoustic measuring device for insert earphones whose acoustic impedance matches that of the average adult ear canal. IEC 60318-4 specifies the device. *See also* ACOUSTIC

COUPLER, ARTIFICIAL EAR, EAR SIMULATOR.

occlusion effect when a sound is present in the ear canal, an increase in the loudness of the sound when the ear canal is blocked (occluded) at its outer end. The effect is most marked at frequencies below 1000 Hz.

occupational hearing loss *see* INDUSTRIAL DEAFNESS.

occupational noise exposure exposure to noise that is experienced by a person when at work. Significant exposure may lead to industrial deafness. *See also* NOISE EXPOSURE LEVEL, NOISE IMMISSION LEVEL.

octave a logarithmic unit of frequency, i.e., a unit of frequency interval, corresponding to an increase in frequency by a factor of two. For example, 50 Hz to 100 Hz is one octave, 125 Hz to 500 Hz is two octaves, etc.

octave band (1) a range of frequency whose upper and lower limits are separated by one octave.

octave band (2) a signal with a bandwidth of one octave.

octave-band analysis analysis of a signal by decomposing it into adjacent octave bands, e.g., bands centred at the preferred frequencies 125, 250, 500 Hz, etc. *See also* OCTAVE FILTER, THIRD-OCTAVE ANALYSIS.

octave filter a bandpass filter whose bandwidth is one octave, i.e., for which the ratio of the upper band-edge frequency to the lower band-edge frequency is 2:1. A set of octave filters covering adjacent frequency ranges can be used for spectrum analysis. Standardised centre frequencies for such octave filters are 125, 250, 500 Hz, etc. *See also* BANDPASS FILTER.

offset error an unwanted positive or negative shift in the readings on an indicator or the signals in a device, for example the output voltage of an amplifier, observed equally across the available range of reading or signal. Also known as zero error, because the error is most apparent when the reading or signal is expected to be zero. *See also* DRIFT.

omnidirectional a term applied to a transducer such as a microphone to indicate that the response of the device is substantially independent of the direction of sound incidence. *See also* DIRECTIONAL MICROPHONE, UNIDIRECTIONAL MICROPHONE.

open-circuit voltage the output voltage of a device measured under conditions of no significant electrical load.

open earmould an earmould which does not significantly occlude the ear canal, used where the outer ear is to be fitted with an earmould but obstructed as little as possible.

open-set test an identification test in which, as far as the subject is aware, there is no restriction on the range of test stimuli, of a given class, which may be presented. The opposite of a closed-set test where a limited number of test items are used and the subject has advance notice of these.

optokinetic nystagmus *see* NYSTAGMUS.

oral by mouth.

oralism the use of the auditory-oral approach to the education of deaf children. This approach is based on the use of speech and the use of residual hearing: the use of sign language is not accepted as an educational means of communication. *See also* TOTAL COMMUNICATION.

oralist a person who subscribes to the auditory-oral approach for the education of deaf children. This approach is based on the use of speech and the use of residual hearing: the use of sign language is not accepted as an educational means of communication.

organ of Corti a major component of the structure that divides the cochlea containing the inner and outer hair cells. *See* Figure 2, under EAR.

orientation the angular position of a person or device relative to a reference direction.

orienting response the response to a sound which involves turning the head towards the direction from which the sound emanates.

oscillation a variation in a parameter such as the position of an object or a signal voltage, up and down in a regular manner.

oscillator a device which produces a periodically varying output, e.g., a sinusoidal motion or a sinusoidal electrical signal.

ossicles the three small bones in the middle ear – malleus, incus and stapes – that connect the eardrum to the oval window of the cochlea, thereby conducting sound from the outer ear to the inner ear. *See* Figure 2, under EAR.

ossicular chain the set of ossicles.

otalgia earache.

otitis inflammation of the ear. *See also* OTITIS EXTERNA, OTITIS MEDIA.

otitis externa inflammation of the outer ear

otitis media inflammation of the middle ear

otoacoustic emission (OAE) an acoustic response produced by the cochlea when stimulated by an acoustic signal, for example, a click or a tonal stimulus. The echo may be picked up by a probe microphone in the ear canal and is generally processed through a computer to average many responses. It is present only where the hearing threshold level is within about 30 dB of normal, and so can be used to identify essentially normal peripheral hearing. Also known as the Kemp echo or an evoked otoacoustic emission (EOAE). *See also* SPONTANEOUS OTOACOUSTIC EMISSION.

otologically normal person a person in a normal state of health who is free from all signs or symptoms of ear disease and from obstructing wax in the ear canal, and who has no history of undue exposure to noise, to potentially ototoxic drugs, or of familial hearing loss (ISO 8253-3).

otologist an ear, nose and throat surgeon specializing in the ear.

otology the science of the ear and ear diseases.

otorhinolaryngologist ear, nose and throat surgeon (ENT surgeon).

otosclerosis a middle ear disease which causes bony growths on the ossicles, in particular the stapes, hence reducing their freedom of movement and causing a conductive hearing loss.

otoscope a device for looking into the ear canal and at the eardrum. Also called an auriscope. *See also* EAR LIGHT

otoscopic examination a visual examination of the ear canal and eardrum by means of an otoscope.

ototoxic drugs drugs that can cause damage to the auditory system, resulting in a hearing loss.

outer ear that part of the ear comprising the pinna and the ear canal. *See* Figure 2, under EAR.

output compression *see* COMPRESSION.

oval window a membrane-covered opening into the cochlea which fits the base of the stapes, allowing transmission of vibration from the middle ear into the inner ear. Also known by its Latin name fenestra ovalis. *See* Figure 2, under EAR.

overall input-related interference level (OIRIL) a parameter used to characterize the immunity of a hearing aid to electromagnetic interference. The OIRIL expresses the interference at the output of the hearing aid as an equivalent acoustic input to the microphone. It is measured with a standardized broadband interference signal. This compares with IRIL which is measured with a 1 kHz pure tone. *See* INPUT-RELATED INTERFERENCE LEVEL.

overload indicator an indicator on a measuring instrument such as a sound level meter, or on an amplifier, etc., which indicates that the input signal has exceeded the range for normal operation. *See also* HEADROOM.

overtone a term used, most often in connection with musical sounds where the sound wave can be decomposed into a discrete set of frequency components, to indicate a component at a frequency higher than the frequency corresponding to the pitch of the sound. The overtones may be labelled first, second, third, etc., in order of ascending frequency. In the case of a sound with a strictly periodic waveform, the first overtone is the second harmonic, the second overtone is the third harmonic, etc. *See also* PARTIAL.

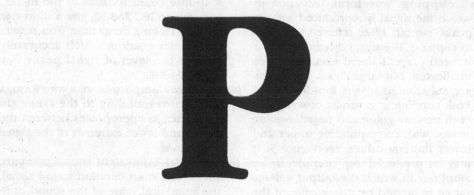

Pa *see* PASCAL.

PA *see* PUBLIC-ADDRESS SYSTEM.

PAM response *see* POST-AURICULAR MYO-GENIC RESPONSE.

PB test *see* PHONEMICALLY BALANCED TEST.

PCM *see* PULSE-CODE MODULATION.

PI *see* PERFORMANCE-INTENSITY FUNCTION.

PPM (in electroacoustics) *see* PEAK PRO-GRAMME METER.

PTS *see* PERMANENT THRESHOLD SHIFT.

paediatric audiology audiology related to the hearing of children.

pain threshold *see* THRESHOLD OF PAIN.

paired comparison a test procedure in which the subject has to compare two test signals (often two alternative versions of the same basic test signal) or a test signal with a reference signal. *See also* METHOD OF ADJUSTMENT, METHOD OF CONSTANT STIMULI.

Palantype a form of machine shorthand in which an operator types on a purpose-designed keyboard. Nowadays combined with electronic processing to provide verbatim transcripts of court-room proceedings and meetings. Used in a 'live' mode to provide on-line transcripts for deaf people. The Stenograph/Stenotype system, used in the USA, and Velotype in Europe are similar.

paracusis the ability of a person with con-ductive hearing loss to understand speech in a noisy environment better than a person with normal hearing.

partial a sinusoidal component of a complex sound wave (IEC 801-30-02). The term is used in cases where the sound wave can be decomposed into a discrete set of frequency components. *See also* HARMONIC, OVERTONE.

pascal the SI (International System) unit of pressure. The symbol is Pa. One pascal (1 Pa) is equivalent to one newton per square metre (1 N m^{-2}) or ten dynes per square centimetre (10 dyne cm^{-2}).

pass band of a filter, the range of frequency over which there is no significant attenuation of input signals. *See also* CUT-OFF FREQUENCY, STOP BAND.

passive transducer a transducer in which the energy of the output signal is derived exclusively from the input signal (IEC 801-25-05), for example, a microphone of a type which can function without an internal battery or other power source. *See also* ACTIVE TRANS-DUCER.

pathology (1) the functional or material changes associated with a disease.

pathology (2) the study of the functional and material changes associated with disease states. *See also* SPEECH PATH-OLOGY.

peak clipping waveform distortion in which the signal is reproduced with its peaks 'cut off', often referred to simply as clipping. The signal dynamic range is limited – small signal excursions are unaffected, but large signal excursions are substituted by the limiting value. Peak clipping is generally observed on both positive-going and negative-going peaks, with corresponding upper and lower limiting values, *see* Figure 5. It may be produced, for example, by an amplifier in which the output voltage range is limited by the voltage of the power supply. In a hearing-aid, circuitry may be included to produce peak clipping at a particular level of the output signal in order to limit the acoustic output. *See also* CENTRE CLIPPING, SATURATION.

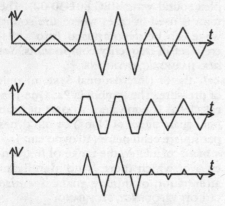

Figure 5. Examples of peak and centre clipping. Upper curve the original waveform; middle curve with peak clipping applied; lower curve with centre clipping applied.

peak level the maximum instantaneous level of a stated kind that occurs during a stated time interval (IEC 801-22-10). *See also* PEAK-TO-PEAK EQUIVALENT SOUND PRESSURE LEVEL, PEAK-TO-PEAK AMPLITUDE.

peak programme meter (PPM) a meter designed for monitoring the level of speech and music in broadcasting and similar audio applications. The time-response characteristics of the meter, specified in IEC 268-10, give a short rise time and a long decay time. This results in a meter reading which accurately reflects the level of signal peaks. *See also* VU METER.

peak-to-peak amplitude of a waveform, a value corresponding to the range (in volts, etc., as appropriate) between the upper and lower extremes of the signal excursions.

peak-to-peak-equivalent sound pressure level of a short-duration sound signal, the numerical value of the sound pressure level (r.m.s) of a long-duration sinusoidal signal which, under the same measurement conditions, has the same peak-to-peak sound pressure as the short duration signal (IEC 60645-3). *See* Figure 6 b).

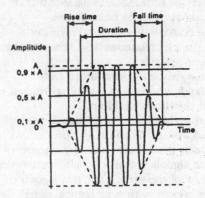

Figure 6 a)

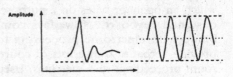

Figure 6 b)

Figure 6. Signals of short duration (IEC 60645-3).
a) Temporal characteristics of a brief tone
b) Waveforms of a click and a peak-to-peak-equivalent sinusoidal signal.

peak-to-peak-equivalent vibratory force level of a short-duration vibratory signal, the numerical value of the vibratory force level (r.m.s.) of a long-duration sinusoidal signal which, under the same measurement conditions, has the same peak-to-peak vibratory force amplitude as the short duration signal (IEC 60645-3). *See* Figure 6 b).

perceived noise level a frequency-weighted sound pressure level in decibels, obtained by a stated procedure that combines the sound pressure levels in the 24 one-third octave bands centred on 50 Hz to 10 kHz (IEC 801-29-11). The algorithm for combining the one-third-octave levels obtained from a particular noise source is intended to produce a figure that corresponds to the subjective noise level. An adjustment may be made to allow for the effect of tonal components in the noise, using an additional algorithm, in which case the quantity is referred to as tone-corrected perceived noise level. *See also* CALCULATED LOUDNESS LEVEL, EFFECTIVE PERCEIVED NOISE LEVEL, JUDGED PERCEIVED NOISE LEVEL, LOUDNESS LEVEL, NOISINESS.

perceptive deafness a lay term for sensorineural deafness.

perfect pitch *see* ABSOLUTE PITCH.

performance-intensity function (PI function) a graph of results from subject testing, plotted as a function of stimulus level. A speech audiogram is an example of a performance-intensity function. *See also* PSYCHOMETRIC FUNCTION.

perilymph fluid that fills the scala vestibuli and scala tympani, similar in composition to the cerebrospinal fluid which bathes the brain.

perinatal in the weeks immediately before and after the birth of a child. *See also* ANTENATAL, POSTNATAL.

period of a repetitive waveform or motion, the time required to complete one cycle, i.e., to return to the same point in the repetition.

periodic repeating regularly. The waveform of a periodic signal consists of a sequence of identical sections, equally spaced along the time axis. *See also* APERIODIC.

periodicity pitch the pitch associated with a complex periodic signal whose spectrum consists of several harmonic components but excludes the fundamental. This pitch corresponds to the frequency of the missing fundamental. For example, components at 450, 600, 750 and 900 Hz will be perceived as having a pitch corresponding to 150 Hz, even though no component at 150 Hz is present in the signal. Also called residue pitch, virtual pitch and low pitch.

peripheral auditory system an inclusive term for the outer ear, the middle ear, the inner ear and the auditory nerve, i.e., that part of the auditory system that precedes the higher neural pathways. Also known as the auditory periphery.

permanent threshold shift (PTS) an increase in hearing threshold level on a permanent basis. Examples of agents that cause PTS include chronic noise exposure and ototoxic drugs. *See also* TEMPORARY THRESHOLD SHIFT – a similar phenomenon whose effects are transitory.

personal sound-exposure meter a wearable sound-level meter that measures both sound pressure and its variation over time in order to establish the sound exposure of an individual over a period of time. Sound exposure is determined as the time integral of the squared, instantaneous A-weighted sound pressure. Such devices are specified in IEC 61252.

personality inventory a psychological test that aims to assess the personality of an individual in terms of a number of traits (e.g., sociability, extroversion, etc.). The assessment is based on the individual's responses to a set of questions.

pharynx the throat; the cavity between the mouth and nose (above) and the joint opening of the gullet and the windpipe (below).

phase (1) for a periodic signal, a quantity

which specifies the timing of signal cycles with respect to the cycles of a reference signal with the same period. (In the reference signal, time zero generally coincides with the start of a cycle.) When measured in radians, a phase θ corresponds to a time advance $T\theta/2\pi$ for the signal waveform, where T is the signal period. Alternatively, when measured in degrees, a phase θ corresponds to a time advance $T\theta/360$ for the signal waveform. The phase will generally lie in the range 0 to 2π radians (or 0 to 360 degrees) since the top of this range corresponds to an advance of a complete period T.

phase (2) a quantity which specifies the timing of an event within the cycle of a periodic signal. When measured in radians, a phase θ corresponds to a time offset $T\theta/2\pi$ from the start of the cycle, where T is the signal period. Alternatively, when measured in degrees, a phase θ corresponds to a time offset of $T\theta/360$ from the start of the cycle. The phase will lie in the range 0 to 2π radians (or 0 to 360 degrees) since the top of this range corresponds to the maximum time offset T.

phase response of a system such as an electronic amplifier or filter, for a given input frequency, the difference between the output phase and the input phase. If the output phase is greater than the input phase, the phase response will be positive; if the output phase is less than the input phase, the phase response will be negative. The phase response is generally measured over a range of frequencies and plotted as a function of frequency. *See also* AMPLITUDE RESPONSE, FREQUENCY RESPONSE, TRANSFER FUNCTION.

phon the unit of loudness level. *See* LOUDNESS LEVEL.

phonation activity of the larynx (involving vocal-cord vibration) to produce a voiced sound, as in the production of a vowel. Also known as vocalization or voicing.

phoneme one of the set of phonemes: the smallest units of sound in a given language that signal a difference between words. For example, the word 'shall' is composed of three phonemes – an initial consonant, a vowel and a final consonant. *See also* MORPHEME.

phoneme scoring in speech audiometry, scoring in terms of percent-correct identification of individual phonemes rather than percent-correct identification of whole words.

phonemic analysis the analysis of speech into a sequence of phonemes, e.g., by manual transcription or by electronic signal processing.

phonemic regression the inability to understand words even though they are heard clearly.

phonemically balanced (PB) test a test of speech recognition in which the frequency of occurrence of the various phonemes in the speech test material is intended to approximate the frequency of occurrence of phonemes in normal speech.

phonetic alphabet a set of letter-like symbols representing the sounds (phonemes) of a particular language. *See also* INTERNATIONAL PHONETIC ALPHABET.

phonetic symbol a letter-like symbol that represents a particular speech sound (phoneme), as specified in the International Phonetic Alphabet.

phonetically balanced test *see* PHONEMICALLY BALANCED TEST, for which the term has been sometimes used.

phonetics *see* ACOUSTIC PHONETICS.

phonology the study of acoustic phonetics.

phonometer an instrument designed to measure subjective loudness. In order to match the variation of the ear's sensitivity with frequency at different levels, a phonometer incorporates filters whose responses correspond to equal-loudness-level contours.

phonophobia an abnormal sense of discomfort brought on by sound above the threshold of hearing.

physiological acoustics the study of the

physiological responses to sound, i.e. mechanical, neural and other physical disturbances.

physiological noise noise of internal origin perceived by a subject when the ear is covered, for example by an earphone. This noise derives from sources such as the subject's heartbeat or may be generated within the ear. *See also* TINNITUS.

pick-up coil *see* INDUCTION COIL (1).

pico the SI prefix denoting 10^{-12}. The abbreviation is p. For example, 5 pW (i.e., 5 picowatts) is 5×10^{-12} watts.

piezoelectric effect the production of a voltage by certain materials when subjected to a mechanical deformation. The effect is reversible – a piezoelectric material will deform when a voltage is applied between opposite faces of a sample.

piezoelectric transducer a transducer in which the conversion from an electrical to a mechanical (acoustic) signal, or vice versa, is performed by a piezoelectric element.

pink noise noise whose spectral distribution is biased towards lower frequencies, with a spectrum level which falls at 3 dB per octave. When applied to a set of constant-percentage-bandwidth analysing filters (e.g., one-third-octave filters), a pink-noise source produces equal power in each filter, since the falloff in spectrum level with increasing frequency is balanced by the increase in bandwidth of the analyser channels. *See also* WHITE NOISE.

pinna that part of the ear that is normally visible. *See* Figure 2, under EAR. Also called the auricle or the external ear.

pistonphone an apparatus having a rigid piston which can be given a reciprocating motion of known frequency and amplitude, so permitting the establishment of a known sound pressure in a closed cavity of small dimensions (IEC 801-28-11). Used to calibrate microphones on sound-level meters. *See also* SOUND CALIBRATOR.

pitch that attribute of auditory sensation in terms of which sounds may be ordered on a scale extending from low to high (IEC 801-29-01). *See also* ABSOLUTE PITCH, MEL, RELATIVE PITCH.

pitch extractor an electronic device or software algorithm for determining the fundamental frequency of voiced speech sounds. With continuous speech as input, the output of a pitch extractor output gives the variation of voice fundamental frequency as a function of time (the intonation pattern) and indicates the time pattern of voicing.

pitch interval *see* INTERVAL.

place of articulation for a particular consonant, the location of the principal vocal-tract movement associated with the production of that consonant. Consonants may be classified according to their place of articulation. For example, the *p* sound is produced by closing the lips and has labial place of articulation. *See also* MANNER OF ARTICULATION.

place theory a model of frequency analysis in the inner ear which assumes a highly localized mechanical response from the basilar membrane to a given frequency, and hence highly localized activation of the hair cells which are distributed along the basilar membrane. Different frequencies activate the hair cells at different places on the basilar membrane – high frequencies close to the basal end of the cochlea and low frequencies close to the apical end. Recent advances in cochlear mechanics have, broadly speaking, tended to confirm the main features of this theory.

placebo a treatment with no active component. Any effect on the patient is thus by suggestion.

plane wave a wave in which the wavefronts are everywhere parallel planes, normal to the direction of propagation (IEC 801-23-06). *See also* CYLINDRICAL WAVE, SPHERICAL WAVE.

play audiometry a form of audiometry used mainly with very young children who cannot undertake conventional audiometry. The child is taught to respond to the test signal by some defined form of play, e.g., by placing a toy figure in a toy boat. *See also* CONDITIONING, GO GAME, TOY TEST, VISUAL-REINFORCEMENT AUDIOMETRY.

playback the reproduction of a previously recorded signal.

plosive *see* STOP (1).

pocket aid *see* BODYWORN AID.

point source (of sound) a source that radiates sound as if from a single point (IEC 801-21-34). The sound field consists of spherical wavefronts, the radius of any particular wavefront increasing with time as energy moves away from the source at the speed of sound.

polar plot a graphical representation of the directional response of a device, e.g., the response of a microphone as a function of the propagation angle of the incident sound. The data are plotted on a circular graph using polar co-ordinates in which the angle co-ordinate corresponds directly to the angle in the experimental situation and the radius co-ordinate corresponds to the magnitude of the response at that angle.

polarization voltage (in acoustics) the voltage which must be applied across the plates of a condenser microphone in order for it to operate.

polarity (1) the attribute – positive or negative – which distinguishes the terminals of a d.c. power supply such as a battery. Terminal polarities indicate the direction of current flow: positive current flows from the positive terminal to the negative terminal.

polarity (2) the attribute – positive or negative – which distinguishes the terminals of an electrical device which operates with a.c. signals, such as a loudspeaker. Terminal-polarity labels can be used to ensure consistent connection of devices of the same type, e.g. the two loudspeakers in a stereo system.

polysyllabic having many syllables. *See also* MONOSYLLABLE.

positional nystagmus *see* NYSTAGMUS.

positive feedback *see* FEEDBACK.

post-aural aid *see* BEHIND-THE-EAR AID.

post-auricular aid *see* BEHIND-THE-EAR AID.

post-auricular myogenic (PAM) response the contraction of a small muscle behind the pinna which is activated by sound, enabling an evoked response to be measured.

post-stimulatory masking *see* FORWARD MASKING.

postlingual deafness deafness whose onset occurs after the acquisition of speech or the ability to understand spoken language. *See also* PRELINGUAL DEAFNESS.

postlingually deaf person someone who becomes deaf after acquiring speech or the ability to understand spoken language. *See also* PRELINGUALLY DEAF PERSON.

postnatal in the period after the birth of a child. *See also* ANTENATAL, PERINATAL.

power amplifier an amplifier designed to deliver power into a low-impedance load, i.e., with the capacity to provide the significant output currents which may be drawn by such a load. The signal from a source with limited capacity to deliver current can be applied to a low-impedance load by way of a power amplifier. (A power amplifier may be contrasted with a voltage amplifier, used to increases the amplitude of a signal voltage, which is not generally intended to deliver significant output power.) *See also* CLASS A, B, C, D, PUSH-PULL AMPLIFIER.

power law the mathematical relationship that exists between two variables, x and y, say, when y varies as x to the power a. This is described by the equation $y = bx^a$, where a and b are constants.

power spectral density the limit, as the bandwidth approaches zero, of sound power divided by bandwidth (IEC 801-21-44). For a given signal with a continuous spectrum, the power spectral density function (i.e., a graph of power spectral density as a function of frequency) indicates the distribution of power with frequency, and is sometimes referred to as the power spectrum of the signal. *See also* SPECTRAL DENSITY (the two terms are often used interchangeably).

power spectrum *see* POWER SPECTRAL DENSITY.

power spectrum density an alternative term for power spectral density.

pre-stimulatory masking *see* BACKWARD MASKING.

precedence effect *see* HAAS EFFECT.

preferred frequencies frequencies recommended for acoustical measurements, given in ISO 266. For measurements in octave bands it is recommended that the bands are geometrically centred on 31.5, 63, 125, 250, 500, 1000, 2000, 4000, 8000 Hz, etc. For measurements in one-third-octave bands it is recommended that the bands are geometrically centred on 31.5, 40, 50, 63, 80, 100, 125 Hz, etc. For meas-urements at single frequencies, in octave steps or one-third octave steps, the same frequencies may be used. Over any decade, the preferred frequencies are approximations, using rational numbers, to a series in exact geometric progression (equal logarithmic intervals). *See also* REFERENCE TEST FREQUENCY.

prelingual deafness deafness whose onset occurs before the acquisition of speech or the ability to understand spoken language. *See also* POSTLINGUAL DEAFNESS.

prelingually deaf person someone who is born deaf or becomes deaf before acquiring speech or the ability to understand spoken language. *See also* POSTLINGUALLY DEAF PERSON.

prenatal in the period before the birth of a child. Also known as antenatal.

presbyacusis hearing loss associated with old age.

pressure a quantity defined as force per unit area. *See also* PASCAL, SOUND PRESSURE.

pressure-gradient microphone a microphone that responds substantially to the gradient of sound pressure (IEC 801-26-04). *See also* PRESSURE MICROPHONE.

pressure microphone a microphone that responds substantially to sound pressure (IEC 801-26-03). *See also* PRESSURE-GRADIENT MICROPHONE.

pressure sensitivity of an electroacoustic transducer for sound reception, for a specified frequency, the quotient V/p of the open-circuit voltage V and the sound pressure p acting on the part of the transducer designed to receive sound (IEC 801-25-53 modified). Also known as voltage sensitivity.

pressure wave *see* COMPRESSIONAL WAVE.

prevalence in a defined human population, the number or proportion of persons with a stated characteristic at a particular time.

primary cell a term used to describe what is commonly called a battery, of the type which cannot be recharged and therefore can be used only once. *See also* SECONDARY CELL.

probe microphone a microphone adapted to explore a sound field without significantly disturbing it (IEC 801-26-10). Also called a probe-tube microphone, since the device usually has a long thin probe in the form of a tube.

probe tone a tone used as a stimulus in a measurement of hearing, for example, in a masking experiment where the probe tone is used to measure the hearing threshold and therefore the effect of the masking signal.

probe-tube microphone *see* PROBE MICROPHONE.

processing time in signal-processing hardware or in auditory perception, the time taken to process a signal to obtain a specified outcome.

profound hearing loss hearing loss which exceeds some 90 dB HL and which results in an inability to hear speech except with the most powerful hearing aids. Even with amplification, a person with a profound hearing loss is unlikely to recognise speech sufficiently well to be able to communicate by hearing alone. A person with a profound hearing loss may be referred to as being profoundly deaf. *See also* AUDIOMETRIC DESCRIPTOR.

profoundly deaf *see* PROFOUND HEARING LOSS.

prognosis a forecast of the progress of a disease or the outcome of treatment.

programmable aid a hearing aid whose performance can be adjusted to fit the needs of the wearer by the use of either a desktop programming unit which is temporarily connected to the aid, or by the use of a control pad which is operated by the wearer.

promontory that part of the middle ear which is between the oval and round windows. *See* Figure 2, under EAR.

proprioception self-awareness of body position and movement.

prosodic features of speech *see* PROSODY, SUPRASEGMENTAL SPEECH FEATURES.

prosody the rhythmic and tonal patterns of speech, corresponding to variations in the intensity, pitch and timing of individual speech elements, over the timescale of words or phrases. Prosodic features can indicate the grouping of speech elements, and features such as stress and inflection. *See also* SUPRASEGMENTAL SPEECH FEATURES.

prosthesis a device intended to compensate for deficiencies in natural function, e.g., a hearing aid, spectacles, etc.

psychoacoustics acoustics relating to auditory perception. *See also* SIGNAL DETECTION THEORY.

psychogalvanic skin response *see* ELECTRODERMAL AUDIOMETRY.

psychogenic deafness *see* NON-ORGANIC HEARING LOSS.

psychometric function a graph of results from subject testing, plotted as a function of a significant stimulus variable. A speech audiogram is an example of a psychometric function. *See also* PERFORMANCE-INTENSITY FUNCTION.

psychosomatic relating to the influence of non-physical stress (fears, emotions, etc.) on the state or function of the body.

public-address system a sound amplification system, used for addressing large assemblies, consisting of microphone(s), amplifier(s) and loudspeaker(s). Often abbreviated to PA system or PA.

pulse a short-duration signal, generally with a clearly defined leading and trailing edge. *See also* BIPHASIC PULSE, MONOPHASIC PULSE.

pulse-code modulation (PCM) a scheme for sending time-varying data – sample values representing a signal waveform – via a digital link which carries a sequence of pulses, modulated to represent a binary code (i.e. each pulse represents a 0 or a 1). Each sample value is converted to a binary number of n bits, say, and the data are sent as blocks of n pulses. Real-time operation is possible, with consecutive blocks (representing consecutive sample values) transmitted at the appropriate rate for the signal waveform to be reconstructed on arrival.

pulse train a sequence of similar but not necessarily identical pulses.

pure tone a sound whose instantaneous sound pressure follows a sinusoidal function of time. Such a sound has only a single frequency component. *See also* SINEWAVE.

pure-tone audiogram *see* AUDIOGRAM.

pure-tone audiometer *see* AUDIOMETER (5).

pure-tone audiometry measurement of hearing with a pure-tone audiometer. *See* AUDIOMETER (5).

push-pull amplifier an amplifier which delivers power to the load via two output devices (e.g. two transistors), one handling positive-going sections of the output signal and the other handling negative-going sections. These devices are generally configured for class-B operation: under no-signal conditions, both devices are 'off' and the current consumption of the circuit is low – a particular advantage of the push-pull design. *See also* POWER AMPLIFIER.

push-to-talk switch a switch on a microphone or telephone which allows the user's voice to be heard only when the switch is operated.

Pythagorean scale a musical scale whose frequency intervals are represented by ratios of integral powers of three and two (IEC 801-30-15), that is, a scale derived from intervals of the octave and the fifth only. *See also* EQUALLY TEMPERED SCALE, JUST SCALE.

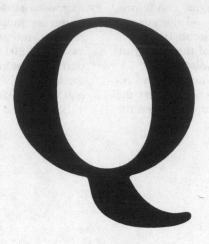

Q a measure of the sharpness of resonance of a system. The higher the *Q*, the
sharper (narrower) the resonance.
There are a variety of mathematical
definitions, but all essentially correspond to the resonant frequency divided by the width in frequency of the
resonant response. Also known as quality factor or *Q* factor. *Note*: Historically,
the letter *Q* was arbitrarily chosen to
designate this quantity. The term quality factor was introduced later.

Q **factor** *see Q*.

quadraphonic a term used to describe
sound reproduction with four loudspeakers to provide spatial distribution
of sound, allowing the listener the sensation of sounds coming from all sides.
See also MONOPHONIC, STEREOPHONIC,
SURROUND SOUND.

quality factor *see Q*.

quasi-free field a sound field that approximates to a free field but is produced by
means other than an anechoic condition. A quasi-free field for audiometric
purposes is specified in ISO 8253-2.

quiescent current the current drawn
from a power supply by an amplifier or
similar circuit under no-signal conditions (i.e., when there is no signal
input and hence no signal output). The
quiescent current may be much less
than the current under signal conditions. For example, a hearing aid may
draw, say, 10 mA at high levels of input
and output, but the quiescent current
may be as low as 500 μA.

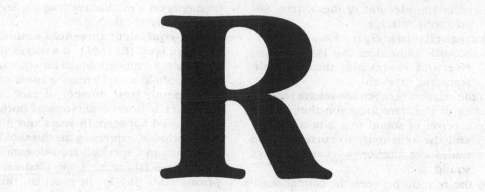

RETFL *see* REFERENCE EQUIVALENT THRESH-
OLD FORCE LEVEL.

RETSPL *see* REFERENCE EQUIVALENT THRESH-
OLD SOUND PRESSURE LEVEL.

Rainville test *see* SENSORINEURAL ACUITY
LEVEL TEST.

random incidence incidence of sound
waves from all directions with equal
probability (IEC 801-31-16). *See also*
RANDOM-INCIDENCE SOUND FIELD.

random-incidence sound field a sound
field consisting of a succession of equal
sound waves incident from all directions with equal probability. *See also*
DIFFUSE SOUND FIELD.

random noise *see* NOISE (1).

rarefaction a reduction in local density,
and hence in local pressure, corresponding to the negative-going part of
an acoustic wavefront. (The positive-
going part of a wavefront is associated
with a compression, i.e., an increase in
local density and local pressure.)

rating scale a scale designed to measure
the subjective impression of an
attribute, e.g., to measure loudness,
quality of sound, etc. by assigning a
number or a given descriptor to the
sound.

Rayleigh disk or **Rayleigh disc** a disk on

a torsion suspension designed to measure the sound particle velocity in a fluid
(IEC 801-28-12).

reactance the component of impedance
corresponding to energy storage (as
opposed to resistance, which is the
component of impedance corresponding to energy dissipation). When using
conventional complex notation, the
reactance is the imaginary part of an
impedance. [This definition applies
when considering electrical impedance,
acoustic impedance, mechanical impedance, etc.]

reaction time the time that a subject takes
to respond, in some defined manner, to
a stimulus. This time has two main components: (i) for central processing, (ii)
for the motor actions required to give
the response.

real-ear measurement a measurement
made on an individual's ear as opposed
to one made in an ear simulator. Measurements in ear simulators do not necessarily produce the same results as
those made on a real ear which are specific to an individual.

receiver (in electroacoustics) a term
used for the earphone in a hearing aid
or telephone, deriving from the fact that

the earphone in a telephone is the receiving element of the system. *See also* BONE VIBRATOR.

reciprocity principle for an electro-acoustic transducer that is linear, passive and reversible, the principle according to which:

a) the relation between the voltage sensitivity of the transducer functioning as a receiver of sound (e.g. a microphone) and the sensitivity to current of the transducer functioning as an emitter of sound, and

b) the relation between the current sensitivity of the transducer functioning as a receiver of sound (e.g. a microphone) and the sensitivity to voltage of the transducer functioning as an emitter of sound, depend only on the geometry of the transducer, the frequency and physical properties of the medium (IEC 801-25-60).

In practice, this means that there is a known relation between the sensitivities of an appropriate transducer (i.e., when used as an emitter and as a receiver) – this provides the basis for the technique of reciprocity calibration for microphones.

recruitment in certain cases of hearing impairment, for example of cochlear origin, an increase in loudness with increasing stimulus magnitude at a rate greater than for a normal ear (IEC 801-29-30).

reference electrode *see* ACTIVE ELECTRODE, INDIFFERENT ELECTRODE.

reference equivalent threshold force level (RETFL) at a specified frequency, the mean value of the equivalent threshold force levels of a sufficiently large number of ears of otologically normal persons of both sexes aged between 18 and 30 years inclusive, expressing the threshold of hearing in a specified mechanical coupler for a specified configuration of bone vibrator (ISO 389-3). In practice, the typical threshold is established in terms of a bone-vibrator drive voltage and this voltage is convert-ed to an equivalent force level by measurements on a mechanical coupler. *See also* AUDIOMETRIC ZERO.

reference equivalent threshold sound pressure level (RETSPL) at a specified frequency, the modal value of the equivalent threshold sound pressure levels of a sufficiently large number of ears of otologically normal persons of both sexes, aged between 18 years and 30 years inclusive, expressing the threshold of hearing in a specified acoustic coupler or artificial ear for a specified earphone (ISO 389-1). In practice, the typical threshold is established in terms of a headphone drive voltage and this voltage is converted to an equivalent sound pressure level by measurements on an ear simulator. *See also* AUDIOMETRIC ZERO, MINIMUM AUDIBLE FIELD.

reference pressure *see* REFERENCE SOUND PRESSURE.

reference sound pressure a sound pressure of 20 μPa, used as the reference in acoustics in air. *See also* DECIBEL, REFERENCE EQUIVALENT THRESHOLD SOUND PRESSURE LEVEL.

reference speech recognition curve for a specified signal and a specified manner of presentation, a curve that describes the median speech recognition score as a function of speech level for a sufficiently large number of otologically normal persons of both sexes, aged between 18 and 25 years inclusive and for whom the test material is appropriate (ISO 8253-3).

reference speech recognition threshold level for a specified speech signal and a specified manner of signal presentation, the median value of the speech recognition threshold levels of a sufficiently large number of otologically normal test persons of both sexes, aged between 18 and 25 years inclusive and for whom the test material is appropriate (ISO 8253-3).

reference test frequency the frequency chosen as standard for making a specific measurement. In the case of hearing aids, 1600 Hz and 2500 Hz are specified. For many purposes 1 kHz is the norm. *See also* PREFERRED FREQUENCIES.

refraction (in acoustics) a phenomenon by which the direction of propagation of a sound wave is changed when the wave encounters a spatial variation in the speed of sound (IEC 801-23-23). *See also* DIFFRACTION.

regression line a line drawn through a scatter plot of paired (x, y) data which mathematically expresses any trend towards a mathematical relationship (usually a linear relationship) between the two variables.

Reissner's membrane the membrane which, together with the basilar membrane, forms the space that contains the endolymph in the cochlea. *See* Figure 2, under EAR.

relative pitch the attribute of a person who can judge the pitch of a musical note accurately and/or can accurately produce a note of a certain pitch on demand, with the aid of a reference against which pitch comparisons can be made. *See also* ABSOLUTE PITCH.

release time in an AGC system, the time taken for the circuit to respond to a sudden decrease of input level, i.e., the time taken to bring up the output level to the appropriate value. *See also* ATTACK TIME.

remote masking the phenomenon by which a noise or tone at relatively high intensity (over some 60 dB SPL), distant in frequency from a test tone, can produce a considerable masking of the test tone.

residual hearing a term used to describe the hearing abilities that remain in a case of severe or profound deafness.

residual inhibition the release from tinnitus which persists for some time after a masking sound has stopped. *See also* TINNITUS MASKER.

residue pitch *see* PERIODICITY PITCH.

resistance the component of impedance corresponding to energy dissipation (as opposed to reactance, which is the com-

ponent of impedance corresponding to energy storage). When using conventional complex notation, the resistance is the real part of an impedance. [This definition applies when considering electrical impedance, acoustic impedance, mechanical impedance, etc.] *See also* ACOUSTIC RESISTANCE, MECHANICAL RESISTANCE.

resonance a phenomenon of a system in forced oscillation such that any change, however small, in the frequency of excitation results in a decrease in the response of the system (IEC 801-24-05). In other words, a resonance corresponds to a peak in the graph of system response versus frequency. *See also* ANTIRESONANCE, Q, RESONANCE FREQUENCY.

resonance frequency a frequency at which there is a peak in the response of a system, i.e., at which a resonance exists. Also known as resonant frequency.

resonant frequency *see* RESONANCE FREQUENCY.

response *see* AMPLITUDE RESPONSE, FREQUENCY RESPONSE, PHASE RESPONSE.

retinitis pigmentosa a degenerative condition of the retina in the eye which occurs in Usher's syndrome, a disease which also affects hearing.

retrocochlear beyond the cochlea (literally, behind the cochlea). A retrocochlear lesion would be a lesion in the auditory pathways after leaving the cochlea but before entering the brainstem, i.e., on the auditory nerve. *See also* SENSORINEURAL HEARING LOSS.

retrospective study study of a phenomenon which, at the time of investigation, has already happened.

reverberant sound field a sound field in which substantially all sound waves have been reflected several times from a boundary of the medium (IEC 801-23-32). Thus reverberant sound dominates, with only a small proportion of the sound coming directly from the source. In a room with a significant amount of reverberation, with a sound source positioned towards the centre of the room, for example, the sound field close to the source will be dominated. by direct sound and the sound field distant from the source will be reverberant.

reverberation sound that persists in a space as a result of repeated reflections or scattering after the source of sound has stopped (IEC 801-21-14). In cases where the sound source is continuous, each time segment of the original sound will persist and hence overlap time-wise with preceding and following segments. *See also* REVERBERATION ROOM, REVERBERATION TIME.

reverberation room a room having long reverberation time, especially designed to make the sound field as diffuse as possible (IEC 801-31-13).

reverberation time of an enclosure, for a sound of a given frequency or frequency band, the time that would be required for the sound pressure level in the enclosure to decrease by 60 decibels, after the source has stopped (IEC 801-31-07). Mostly applied to rooms, where reverberation times in particular ranges are desirable for applications such as music performance, public speaking etc. *See also* DECAY TIME.

reversible transducer a transducer capable of transforming an electrical signal into an acoustic or mechanical signal, and the converse (IEC 801-25-07). For example, although not designed for the purpose, a moving-coil loudspeaker can act as a microphone.

ribbon microphone a moving-conductor microphone in which the conductor is a thin ribbon and is driven directly by the sound waves (IEC 801-26-18).

Rinne test a bone conduction test undertaken with a tuning fork, where the fork is placed on the mastoid process for a few seconds and then transferred to the opening of the ear canal. In normally hearing subjects the air-conducted sound is heard for longer and is louder. In the case of a conductive hearing loss the bone-conducted sound is heard for longer and is louder. *See also* BING TEST, TUNING-FORK TESTS, WEBER TEST.

rise time the characteristic time duration associated with a process in which some quantity increases systematically with time, tending towards a final value. *See also* DECAY TIME.

roll-off a progressive reduction in response with frequency. [The term generally indicates a gradual fall-off, as opposed to a sharp cut-off at a particular frequency.] *See also* DECIBELS PER OCTAVE, DECIBELS PER DECADE.

root-mean-square amplitude a measure of the amplitude of a signal, equal to the square root of the mean-square value of the signal, this mean-square value being obtained by averaging over a suitable time window.

round window an aperture in the cochlea, situated in the scala tympani. *See* Figure 2, under EAR. Also known by its Latin name fenestra rotunda.

rubella the medical term for German measles. Rubella contracted by a mother in the first months of pregnancy may cause hearing loss and other defects in the child.

running speech a term to used to indicate continuous speech, as is sometimes used for test purposes. *See also* CONNECTED-DISCOURSE TRACKING.

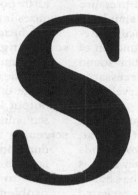

S the symbol used to indicate one of the standard time weightings, Slow, used in sound level meters. *See* TIME WEIGHTING.

'S' indicator an instrument used to show the presence of the speech sound *s* for therapy purposes.

SAL test *see* SENSORINEURAL ACUITY LEVEL TEST.

SAW *see* SURFACE ACOUSTIC WAVE.

SHM *see* SIMPLE HARMONIC MOTION.

SI units units in the Système International d'Unité, the standard units for scientific purposes. The seven base units include the metre, kilogram, second and ampere. They are combined in various ways to form derived units, e.g., the unit of velocity: $m\ s^{-1}$. Several derived units have special names, e.g., newton ($kg\ m\ s^{-2}$), pascal ($kg\ m^{-1}\ s^{-2}$), hertz (s^{-1}).

SISI test *see* SHORT INCREMENT SENSITIVITY INDEX TEST.

SL *see* DECIBEL, SENSATION LEVEL.

SNR *see* SIGNAL-TO-NOISE RATIO.

SONAR *see* SONAR.

SPL *see* DECIBEL, SOUND PRESSURE LEVEL.

SRT *see* SPEECH RECOGNITION THRESHOLD LEVEL.

SSE *see* SIGN SUPPORTED ENGLISH.

SSPL *see* SATURATION SOUND PRESSURE LEVEL.

sabin the unit of Sabine absorption, i.e., of sound absorption as defined by the Sabine reverberation-time equation.

When using SI units, the sabin is generally referred to as the metric sabin. Since the dimensions of sound absorption are those of area, a measurement in metric sabins is often given simply in units of m^2. (When the unit of length is the foot, the sabin corresponds to 1 ft^2 and is thus equal to 0.0929 metric sabins.) *See also* SABINE REVERBERATION-TIME EQUATION.

Sabine absorption *see* SABINE REVERBERATION-TIME EQUATION.

Sabine absorption coefficient for a surface, the Sabine absorption of the surface divided by the area of the surface.

Sabine reverberation-time equation for a room, a theoretical relation between the reverberation time T, the volume V, the total Sabine absorption A (representing absorption of sound at surfaces in the room) and the speed of sound c. For metric units the relation is as follows:

$$T = 55.3\ V/Ac$$

saturation the condition in which the signal at a particular point in an electronic circuit is at the upper or lower limit of the signal range available at that point, this range being determined by the circuit design. *See also* PEAK CLIPPING.

saturation sound pressure level (SSPL)

the highest possible sound pressure level obtainable in an ear simulator from a hearing aid at a specified frequency (or expressed as a function of frequency). *Note:* The saturation sound pressure level does not necessarily occur at the highest input level. (IEC 60118-0). *See also* $OSPL_{90}$.

savart a logarithmic unit of frequency, i.e., a unit of frequency interval. One savart is the interval between two sounds whose fundamental-frequency ratio is the thousandth root of ten. The savart is rarely used – the cent is the preferred unit for small intervals or small changes in interval.

sawtooth wave a signal whose waveform resembles the outline of teeth on a saw, consisting of repeated sections, each with a linear rise followed by a sudden fall (or a linear fall followed by a sudden rise). *See also* SINEWAVE, SQUARE WAVE, TRIANGULAR WAVE.

scala media *see* COCHLEAR DUCT.

scala tympani part of the cochlea that forms a fluid-filled cavity on one side of the basilar membrane and is continuous with the scala vestibuli at the helicotrema. *See* Figure 2, under EAR.

scala vestibuli part of the cochlea that forms a fluid-filled cavity on one side of the basilar membrane and is continuous with the scala tympani at the helicotrema. *See* Figure 2, under EAR.

scalar quantity a quantity that is completely characterized by its magnitude, such as mass, pressure, etc. (as opposed to a vector quantity, such as force, that is characterized by a magnitude and a direction).

scattering reflection and/or diffraction of an incident wave into outgoing waves in many directions.

screened lead a cable of coaxial construction with a centre conductor surrounded by insulation and then by an outer metal screen, usually of metal strands. The term is generally reserved for cables of this type which are designed for use at audio frequencies. With the screen at earth potential, this construction minimizes interference pick-up on the inner conductor. *See also* COAXIAL CABLE.

screening audiometer a pure-tone audiometer, equipped for air-conduction measurements only, with a limited range of measurement frequencies and output levels, designed to be used for screening purposes.

screening test (in audiometry) a short-duration test designed for evaluation of large numbers of individuals with a view to identifying those with hearing problems. A predetermined hearing level is generally set, and subjects pass or fail according to whether or not they respond to the test signal. No attempt is made to measure at any other hearing level or to find the threshold of hearing of the individual.

secondary cell a cell, i.e., an electrical power source, which is designed to be recharged after it has been used. *See also* PRIMARY CELL.

segmental speech features features of speech which occur on the timescale of a phoneme. As opposed to suprasegmental speech features which occur on a longer timescale.

self noise *see* INHERENT NOISE.

self-recording audiometer *see* AUDIOMETER (4).

self-recording audiometry audiometry using an automatic-recording audiometer.

semantics the study of meaning of words and the development of meanings.

semi-vowel *see* MANNER OF ARTICULATION.

semicircular canals the structure containing the vestibular system, i.e., the sense organ of balance, consisting of three canals which are mutually perpendicular, forming part of the inner ear. *See* Figure 2, under EAR.

semitone the smallest interval used in conventional Western music. On many musical instruments the semitone is standardized as an equally tempered semitone, corresponding to a fundamental-frequency ratio of the twelfth root of two. *See also* EQUALLY TEMPERED SCALE.

sensation level (SL) for an individual listener and a specified sound, the amount by which a sound pressure level exceeds the threshold of hearing for that sound (IEC 801-29-29). *See also* DECIBEL.

sensitivity of a transducer, the quotient of a specified quantity describing the output signal of a transducer and another specified quantity describing the corresponding input signal. (IEC 801-25-10 modified). For example, the sensitivity of a microphone might be expressed as 3.5×10^{-3} V Pa^{-1}.

sensitivity level of a transducer, the output level of a stated kind minus the input level of a stated kind that caused the output level. *Note*: The reference values for the input and output levels determine the reference sensitivity and should be chosen accordingly (IEC 801-25-12). In other words, the sensitivity level of a transducer is the sensitivity expressed in decibels. For example, the sensitivity level of a microphone might be expressed as -49 dB *re* 1 V Pa^{-1}.

sensorineural acuity level test (SAL test) a hearing test where masking noise is presented though a bone vibrator, with the test tone being delivered through an earphone, as opposed to the normal method which is the reverse of this, in order to determine the level of conductive hearing loss in difficult-to-test cases. Also known as the Rainville test.

sensorineural hearing loss a hearing loss which relates to the cochlea and/or auditory neural pathways but not to the conductive mechanism of the ear or to the auditory cortex. *See also* RETRO-COCHLEAR, CENTRAL AUDITORY DYSFUNC-TION, CONDUCTIVE HEARING LOSS.

sensory-neural a former spelling of sensorineural.

service life the lifetime of a device, specified in terms of the period over which the device can be appropriately maintained. *See also* SHELF LIFE.

servomechanism a mechanism which automatically adjusts itself in response to changing conditions.

seventh cranial nerve *see* FACIAL NERVE.

severe hearing loss *see* AUDIOMETRIC DESCRIPTOR.

shear wave a wave propagating in an elastic medium that causes an element of the medium to change its shape without a change of volume (IEC 801-23-10). In other words, a wave which travels by virtue of shear forces within the medium, as opposed, for example, to a compressional wave.

shelf life the length of time a device can be kept as new before it is put into operation, particularly relevant to batteries. *See also* SERVICE LIFE.

short-duration signal (in audiometry) a signal having a duration of less than 200 ms (IEC 60645-4). Reference signals of short duration for audiometric and neuro-otological purposes are defined in IEC 60645-4. *See also* BRIEF TONE, FILTERED CLICK, PULSE.

short increment sensitivity index test (SISI test) a test of recruitment in which subjects are required to detect 200 ms increments (magnitude 1 to 5 dB) introduced into a continuous tone.

shot noise electrical noise observed in association with low-value electrical currents, relating to the fact that the discrete nature of electric charge does not allow perfectly steady currents. *See also* INHERENT NOISE, THERMAL NOISE.

sibilants high-frequency fricative speech sounds such as *s*.

sideband a band of frequencies in the spectrum of an amplitude-modulated or frequency-modulated signal, whose characteristics derive from the modulating signal. Sidebands generally occupy the frequency regions immediately above and below the carrier frequency.

sidetone a term used in telephony to describe the effect of a speaker hearing his/her voice from the telephone earpiece.

sign language a language which carries its

information and meaning by means of hand, facial and body movements. Sign language has its own syntax and varies from country to country in the same way that spoken language does. It may be presented with one hand (as in the USA) or with two hands (as in the UK). In the UK the native sign language is known as British Sign Language (BSL). In the USA the native sign language is known as American Sign Language (ASL). *See also* MAKATON, SIGNED ENGLISH.

sign supported English (SSE) a system in which manual signs are synchronized with corresponding spoken words but, in contrast to signed English, these signs cover only a subset of the spoken elements.

signal a variation in time of some quantity so as to carry information or meaning, or in a manner which in principle permits information or meaning to be carried.

signal-detection theory a theoretical analysis of the detection and discrimination of signals by an observer, involving a statistical description of the limits to perception and of the variation in the observer's responses. *See also* PSYCHO-ACOUSTICS.

signal-to-noise ratio (SNR) the ratio of signal amplitude to noise amplitude in a particular situation. When the signal amplitude or noise amplitude are time-varying, it may be convenient to use root-mean-square values. The signal and noise may be acoustic (e.g., when someone is speaking) or electrical (e.g., the output of an amplifier). A high signal-to-noise ratio is generally sought after, since this corresponds to little interference to the signal from the noise. The SNR is often expressed in dB as $20\log_{10}$(signal amplitude/noise amplitude). *See also* SPEECH INTERFERENCE LEVEL.

signed English a system in which manual signs are synchronized with corresponding spoken English to represent the language with full respect to its grammatical constructs. *See also* SIGN SUPPORTED ENGLISH.

silence the absence of audible sound.

simple harmonic motion (SHM) for a body subject to a force proportional to its displacement from equilibrium, this force being directed so as to restore the body to its equilibrium position, the motion that results when the body is displaced from equilibrium and then released. For example, the motion of a mass suspended on an ideal spring. In simple harmonic motion the displacement of the body is a sinusoidal function of time. *See also* SINEWAVE.

simulated in-situ gain *see* IN-SITU GAIN.

sinewave or **sine wave** a signal or wave having the same graphical representation as a sine function, i.e., having only a single frequency component. *See also* PURE TONE, SAWTOOTH WAVE, SQUARE WAVE, TRIANGULAR WAVE.

sinusoidal in the form of a sinewave.

six-cc coupler (often written as **6 cc coupler**) a colloquial reference to the acoustic coupler specified in IEC 303 (now IEC 60318-3) for measurement of the acoustic output of supra-aural earphones. The coupler has a cavity of approximately six cubic centimetres in front of the measuring microphone, hence '6 cc'. *See also* ACOUSTIC COUPLER.

ski-slope hearing loss hearing loss in which hearing is near normal up to a frequency of 1 kHz or more and then falls very rapidly, often to no measurable hearing at frequencies above 4 kHz. The term comes from the shape of the pure-tone audiogram, which looks like a steep ski slope.

social noise noise produced in the course of normal domestic and pleasure activities, e.g., noise from lawnmowers. *See also* AMBIENT NOISE.

socioacusis hearing loss attributable to the damaging effects of noise in everyday normal life, excluding noise at work.

Sona-Graph *see* SOUND SPECTROGRAPH.

sonagram *see* SOUND SPECTROGRAPH.

sonar (SONAR) sound navigation and ranging system used in the underwater detection and location of objects.

sone a unit of loudness, equal to the loudness of a pure tone presented frontally as a plane wave of frequency 1000 Hz and a sound pressure level of 40 dB re 20 μPa. *Note*: The loudness of a sound that is judged by the listener to be *n* times that of the 1-sone tone is *n* sones (IEC 801-29-04). *See also* LOUDNESS LEVEL.

sonic (1) pertaining to sound.

sonic (2) pertaining to the speed of sound.

sonic boom a sound produced when an object, such as a projectile or an aircraft, travels through the air at a speed greater than the local speed of sound.

sonoluminescence the emission of light associated with cavitation in liquids.

sonometer an instrument used for the comparison of frequencies, having a single wire string stretched along a soundbox and an adjustable bridge to change the sounding length of the string. Nowadays used only as a laboratory demonstration.

sound (1) an oscillation of particles in a medium, mediated by elastic forces within the medium.

sound (2) a sensation of hearing evoked by an acoustic oscillation. Often specified by the term audible sound.

sound absorption the process by which sound energy is dissipated (i.e., converted to another form of energy, usually heat) as sound passes through an acoustic medium or reflects from a surface at the boundary of a medium. Absorption results in a reduction of sound level. Also known as acoustic absorption.

sound absorption coefficient (of a surface) the fraction of sound energy absorbed at a specific frequency when a sound wave reflects from a surface.; usually specified for a diffuse sound field. Also known as acoustic absorption coefficient. *See also* SOUND ATTENUATION COEFFICIENT, SABINE ABSORPTION COEFFICIENT.

sound analyser *see* FREQUENCY ANALYSIS, SPECTRUM ANALYSER.

sound attenuation the process by which sound energy is lost from a sound beam as it passes through a medium, either by dissipation (i.e., conversion to heat energy) or by scattering. Also known as acoustic attenuation.

sound attenuation coefficient of a medium, a parameter that describes the rate of fall-off in intensity of a sound beam as a function of distance, due to attenuation processes. Generally expressed in units of decibels per metre (dB m^{-1}). Also known as acoustic attenuation coefficient. *See also* SOUND ABSORPTION COEFFICIENT.

sound balance a term used in recording and broadcasting studios to describe the task of adjusting the levels and characteristics of sounds from different sources to give the required result when these sounds are heard in combination. The term is also used to describe the settings and adjustments used in a particular case.

soundbite a term used in the media to denote a short speech recording which, of its nature, contains little detailed information.

sound calibrator a device used for the calibration of microphones. Sound calibrators are designed to produce a known sound pressure level at a specified frequency when coupled to specified models of microphones in specified configurations. The requirements for sound calibrators are described in IEC 60942. *See also* PISTONPHONE.

sound energy flux density *see* SOUND INTENSITY.

sound exposure a quantity intended to represent the total sound energy received by the ear over a stated time interval or a stated event, such as an aircraft flyover. The sound exposure is the time integral, over the interval or event, of the squared instantaneous sound pressure. The sound pressure is generally A-frequency-weighted, but other frequency weightings may be used. *See also* NOISE EXPOSURE.

sound exposure level sound exposure expressed in decibels; calculated using the formula $10\log_{10}$(sound exposure/reference exposure). The reference exposure is usually taken as 4×10^{-10} Pa^2 s, corresponding to a pressure of 20 μPa integrated over 1 s. *See also* EFFECTIVE PERCEIVED NOISE LEVEL, NOISE EXPOSURE LEVEL.

sound field the region of an elastic medium containing sound waves (IEC 801-23-27). *See also* DIFFUSE SOUND FIELD, FREE SOUND FIELD, RANDOM-INCIDENCE SOUND FIELD, REVERBERANT SOUND FIELD.

sound-field audiometry audiometry which is undertaken using a loudspeaker as the source of sound rather than earphones. The procedures for sound-field audiometry are described in ISO 8253-2.

sound insulation (1) an element in the construction of a wall or partition, intended to prevent the transmission of sound – also known as acoustic insulation. The same term (see next entry) is used to describe the performance of such an element – also known as transmission loss or sound reduction index.

sound insulation (2) of a partition, for a specified frequency band, the difference in decibels between the average sound pressure levels in the reverberant source and receiving rooms, plus ten times the logarithm to the base ten of the ratio of the area of the common partition to the total Sabine absorption in the receiving room (IEC 801-31-39). Also known as transmission loss or sound reduction index.

sound intensity for a sound wave, the average rate of energy flow per unit area, where the area under consideration is normal to the direction of propagation of the wave. Also called acoustic intensity, sound energy flux density, sound power density.

sound intensity level sound intensity expressed in decibels, calculated using the formula $10\log_{10}$(sound intensity/reference intensity). The reference intensity is generally taken as 1 pW m^{-2}.

sound level weighted sound pressure, i.e., sound pressure obtained using a standard frequency weighting and a standard exponential time weighting, expressed in decibels using the formula $20\log_{10}$(weighted sound pressure/reference pressure). The reference pressure is generally taken as 20 μPa. Also known as weighted sound pressure level. *See also* SOUND PRESSURE LEVEL, SOUND INTENSITY LEVEL.

sound level meter an instrument for the measurement of sound level with a standard frequency weighting and a standard exponential time weighting (IEC 801-28-01). The requirements for sound level meters are described in IEC 651.

sound power sound energy per unit time, for example, radiated by a source or crossing an area.

sound power density *see* SOUND INTENSITY.

sound power level sound power expressed in decibels, calculated using the formula $10\log_{10}$(sound power/reference power). The reference power is generally taken as 1 pW.

sound pressure (1) at a point in a medium which carries a sound, the difference between the pressure existing at the time under consideration and the equilibrium pressure. In other words, the component of the pressure which is associated with the sound wave. Also known as acoustic pressure or sometimes [*see* SOUND PRESSURE (2), below] as instantaneous sound pressure.

sound pressure (2) The root-mean-square value of the quantity defined in (1), above. If the term sound pressure is used to indicate such a root-mean-square value, the quantity defined in (1), above, may be referred to as instantaneous sound pressure.

sound pressure level (SPL) sound pressure, usually a root-mean-square value, expressed in decibels using the formula $20\log_{10}$(sound pressure/reference pressure). The reference pressure is generally taken as 20 μPa for airborne sound and 1 μPa for sound in media other than air. *See also* DECIBEL, SOUND LEVEL.

sound reduction index *see* SOUND INSULATION.

sound spectrogram *see* SOUND SPECTROGRAPH.

sound spectrograph an instrument that measures and displays the time-varying spectrum of a sound, mainly used to analyse speech signals (hence also known as a speech spectrograph). The output is in the form of a graphic, known as a spectrogram, in which frequency is represented on the ordinate, time on the abscissa and intensity by grey scale (i.e., the darkness of the image). A commercial instrument of this type is the Sona-Graph, whose output is often referred to as a sonagram. When used for purposes of speaker identification or comparison, the output of a sound spectrograph is sometimes referred to as a voiceprint.

sound spectrum *see* SPECTRUM.

soundboard a wooden board with which a vibrating object such as a tuning fork may be placed in contact, causing the acoustic output of the vibrating object to be enhanced. In a musical instrument such as a piano the soundboard carries the bridge, which in turn carries the strings, and its function is to convert vibrations of the strings into an acoustic output. Also known as a sounding board.

sounding board *see* SOUNDBOARD.

Sparton a manual means of communication used with deaf-blind people. Letters (upper case, i.e., capitals) are traced on the palm of the hand with a finger.

speaking tube an open-ended, air-filled tube used to convey speech from one place to another by channelling the sound generated by the talker. The talker speaks near to one end of the tube and the listener places an ear near to the other end. Used in the past to communicate between different parts of ships or buildings, and also used as an aid for hearing impaired people, in which case the tube is generally flexible and fitted with an ear pip for the listener.

spectacle aid a hearing aid in which all the components are housed in the side arm, or arms, of a pair of spectacles. The aid may have an air-conduction or a bone-conduction output. The American term is eyeglass aid. *See also* HEADBAND AID.

spectral density the limit, as the bandwidth approaches zero, of the mean-square value of a field quantity divided by the bandwidth. The kind of field quantity must be specified, such as sound pressure, particle velocity, particle acceleration. (IEC 801-21-43). Spectral density is the quantity that is used, plotted as a function of frequency, to represent a continuous spectrum, i.e., the spectrum of a signal which has energy continuously distributed with frequency. Also called spectrum density. *See also* POWER SPECTRAL DENSITY (the two terms are often used interchangeably).

spectral density level *see* SPECTRUM LEVEL.

spectrogram *see* SOUND SPECTROGRAPH.

spectrograph *see* SOUND SPECTROGRAPH.

spectrum a representation of the distribution of energy with frequency for a signal, i.e., indicating the magnitudes of the components as a function of frequency. *See also* CONTINUOUS SPECTRUM, LINE SPECTRUM.

spectrum analyser (in acoustics) an apparatus for the determination of the spectrum of a sound, i.e., the distribution of energy with frequency. The distribution is usually measured by filtering the signal into narrow frequency bands. Instruments are often described in terms of the bandwidth of the filters used or the method of analysis, e.g., one-third-octave analyser, FFT analyser, etc. Also known as a sound analyser. *See also* FREQUENCY ANALYSIS.

spectrum density *see* SPECTRAL DENSITY.

spectrum density level *see* SPECTRUM LEVEL.

spectrum level spectral density expressed in decibels, calculated using the formula $10\log_{10}$(spectral density/reference spectral density). The reference spectral density is taken to be the square of the reference amplitude (e.g., for sound pressure, the square of 20 μPa) divided by the reference bandwidth of 1 Hz. For practical purposes, the spectrum level at a given frequency can be taken as the signal level in a 1 Hz band centred at that frequency. Also known as spectral density level or spectrum density level.

specula for ear canal inspection, cone-shaped fittings on an otoscope which may be inserted into the ear canal. (The singular form is speculum.)

specular reflection reflection from a surface in the same manner that light reflects from a mirror, i.e., with the angle of reflection equal to the angle of incidence.

speech and language therapist a therapist who deals with all aspects of defective speech production, including language aspects. This term has now largely replaced the title speech therapist. *See also* HEARING THERAPIST.

speech audiogram *see* AUDIOGRAM.

speech audiometer *see* AUDIOMETER (6).

speech audiometry the technique wherein standardized samples of a language are presented through a calibrated system to measure some aspect of hearing ability (Carhart 1951). *See* AUDIOMETER (6) and Figure 1 c), under AUDIOGRAM.

speech awareness threshold *see* SPEECH DETECTION THRESHOLD LEVEL.

speech detection threshold level for a given test subject, a specified speech signal and a specified manner of signal presentation, the speech level of the test material at which it is detected (but not necessarily understood) in a specified percentage of trials, usually 50%. *Note*: Speech detection threshold has been called speech awareness threshold (ISO 8253-3). *See also* DETECTION THRESHOLD, SPEECH RECOGNITION THRESHOLD LEVEL, THRESHOLD OF HEARING.

speech discrimination score *see* SPEECH RECOGNITION SCORE.

speech hearing level *see* HEARING LEVEL FOR SPEECH.

speech interference level a quantity intended to indicate the potential of background noise to interfere with speech communication. The speech interference level is the arithmetical mean of the sound pressure levels in octave bands centred on 500 Hz, 1000 Hz, 2000 Hz and 4000 Hz, measured at the listener's position during typical noise conditions. *See also* SIGNAL-TO-NOISE RATIO.

speech level the sound pressure level or vibratory force level of a speech signal as measured (with specified frequency weighting and specified time weighting) in an appropriate acoustic or mechanical coupler, artificial ear or in a sound field. For example, the speech level may be expressed as the equivalent continuous sound pressure level or vibratory force level determined by integration over the duration of the speech signal, with frequency weighting C. For speech lists based on single items separated by silent intervals, the integration should not include these intervals. For test lists based on single test items with carrier phrase, the integration should include the test item only (ISO 8253-3). *See also* HEARING LEVEL FOR SPEECH.

speech pathology the study of impaired speech production.

speech reading *or* **speechreading** *see* LIP READING.

speech reception threshold *see* SPEECH RECOGNITION THRESHOLD LEVEL.

speech recognition curve for a specified speech signal and a specified manner of presentation, a curve that describes for an individual test subject the speech recognition score as a function of speech level. *Note*: The speech recognition curve has been called the articulation function (ISO 8253-3).

speech recognition score for a given test subject, a specified speech signal, a specified manner of signal presentation and at a specified speech level, the percentage of correctly recognized test items or scoreable items if the scoring method is not based on whole test items. *Note*: Speech recognition score has been called speech discrimination score (ISO 8253-3). *See also* DISCRIMINATION SCORE, SPEECH RECOGNITION THRESHOLD LEVEL.

speech recognition threshold level for a given test subject, a specified speech signal and a specified manner of signal presentation, the lowest speech level at which the recognition score is equal to 50%. *Note:* Speech recognition threshold has been called speech reception threshold or SRT (ISO 8253-3). *See also* DISCRIMINATION THRESHOLD, SPEECH DETECTION THRESHOLD LEVEL, SPEECH RECOGNITION SCORE.

speech spectrogram *see* SOUND SPECTROGRAPH.

speech spectrograph *see* SOUND SPECTROGRAPH.

speech synthesis production of artificial human speech, i.e., without recourse to the use of recordings of any part of real speech. Speech-synthesis systems involve rule-based models of the speech production process, derived from the study of real speech. The resulting speech is known as synthetic speech. *See also* SYNTHESISER.

speech therapist *see* SPEECH AND LANGUAGE THERAPIST.

speech tracking *see* CONNECTED-DISCOURSE TRACKING.

speech trainer *see* AUDITORY TRAINING UNIT.

spherical wave a wave of which the wave fronts are concentric spheres (IEC 801-23-07).). A spherical wave is emitted by a point source or by a source with spherical symmetry. *See also* CYLINDRICAL WAVE, PLANE WAVE.

spondee a two-syllable word with stress on each syllable, for example, 'bamboo'. Single words used for measurement of speech recognition are generally chosen as monosyllables, spondees or trochees.

square wave a repetitive signal whose waveform switches alternately between two different fixed values, the transitions occurring at equal time intervals and having negligible duration. *See also* SINEWAVE, SAWTOOTH WAVE, TRIANGULAR WAVE.

squelch effect in a situation in which there are two competing sounds, the effect by which a listener is able, by concentrating on one sound, to produce an apparent reduction in the level of the other sound. [This use of the term derives from radio-communications usage, where 'squelch' refers to automatic shut-off of reception when no signal is received, in order to avoid a receiver output with undue levels of background noise.]

standard microphone a microphone whose response is determined accurately by means of a primary calibration method (IEC 801-26-02). Such a microphone can be used for comparison purposes against other microphones.

standard musical pitch a standard musical tuning frequency of 440 Hz for A in the treble stave.

standard a document, established by consensus and approved by a recognized body, that provides, for common or repeated use, rules, guidelines or characteristics for activities or their results, aimed at the achievement of the optimum degree of order in a given context. *Note:* Standards should be based on the consolidated results of science, technology and experience, and aimed at the the promotion of optimum community benefits (BS 0).

standing wave a wave in which the oscillation has a fixed distribution in space, characterized by nodes (positions at which the oscillation amplitude is zero) and antinodes (positions at which the oscillation amplitude is maximum). A standing wave may be produced by the interference of progressive waves propagating in opposite directions. Also known as a stationary wave. *See also* TRAVELLING WAVE.

stapedectomy a surgical operation performed in cases where the movement of the stapes has been restricted by otosclerosis, resulting in a conductive hearing loss. The stapes is removed and replaced by an artificial substitute, for example, a Teflon piston. This allows the vibration associated with sound at the eardrum to be transmitted to the cochlea.

stapedius reflex *see* ACOUSTIC REFLEX.

stapes the last bone in the ossicular chain which conducts vibrations into the cochlea. *See* Figure 2, under EAR.

startle reflex an involuntary movement which may be made by a person in response to a sudden sound or a tactile stimulus.

static pressure *see* EQUILIBRIUM PRESSURE.

stationary wave *see* STANDING WAVE.

steady-state condition an operating condition of a device or system in which there is no change with time.

Stenger test a test in which two tones of the same frequency but different intensity are presented simultaneously, one to each ear of the subject. Only one tone is generally perceived – the more intense tone in the case of a normally hearing subject. The test is used to investigate a suspected non-organic unilateral hearing loss.

Stenograph or **Stenotype** a form of machine shorthand in which an operator types on a purpose-designed phonemic keyboard to input a transcription of what is being said. Nowadays combined with electronic processing to provide verbatim transcripts of courtroom proceedings and meetings. Used in a 'live' mode to provide on-line transcripts for deaf people. The Stenotype system is widely used in the USA. Similar to the Palantype system, used in the UK, and the Velotype system in Europe.

stereo a prefix derived from the Greek word meaning solid, thereby implying three dimensions. *See also* STEREOPHONIC.

stereophonic a term used to describe a sound system with two channels, including separately driven loudspeakers or headphones, giving an impression of spatially distributed sound sources when used for reproduction of a recording. Often abbreviated to stereo. *See also* MONOPHONIC, QUADRAPHONIC, SURROUND SOUND.

stimulus an input intended to provoke a response from a subject. In the case of audiometry the stimulus may be a pure tone, a click or a speech signal.

stop (1) a short consonant whose production involves a sudden release of the air pressure retained behind an occlusion in the vocal tract, e.g., *p* as in 'pie'. Also known as a plosive or stop consonant. For an unvoiced stop such as *p*, the vocal cords do not vibrate; for a voiced plosive such as *b*, vocal-cord vibration (i.e., phonation) contributes an additional component to the sound. *See also* MANNER OF ARTICULATION.

stop (2) to close a hole or finger a string on a musical instrument so as select the required pitch.

stop (3) a set of pipes on an organ, or a device which brings into operation a given set of pipes.

stop band of a filter, the range of frequency over which there is significant attenuation of input signals. *See also* PASS BAND, CUT-OFF FREQUENCY.

sub-threshold below the perceptual threshold. Also known as subliminal. *See also* SUPRATHRESHOLD.

subharmonic a frequency component which may be generated in a system, at an integral sub-multiple of the fundamental frequency of the input signal. For example, an input with a fundamental frequency of 480 Hz may generate subharmonics at 240 Hz, 160 Hz, 120 Hz, etc. *See also* HARMONIC.

subjective audiometry audiometry that involves a test subject who is required to make an overt response. As opposed to objective testing, where the response from the subject is obtained by some form of physiological measurement.

subliminal *see* SUB-THRESHOLD.

subsonic (1) having a speed less than the speed of sound.

subsonic (2) *see* INFRASOUND.

substitution method of measurement a method for determining the sound pressure level at the location of a test object, involving measurement of the sound pressure level at the test point (with a calibrated microphone) without the test object being in place. When the test object is subsequently placed at the test point, the sound pressure at the test object is taken to be that previously measured.

sudden deafness a severe or profound hearing loss with a very short onset period (a few hours to a few days). Such cases requires urgent specialist attention. Also known as sudden hearing loss.

sudden hearing loss *see* SUDDEN DEAFNESS.

summation tone an additional tone present at the output of a non-linear system when two tones are applied to the input, whose frequency is equal to the sum of the two input frequencies. For example, inputs at 100 Hz and 320 Hz can produce a summation tone at 420 Hz. *See also* COMBINATION TONE, DIFFERENCE TONE.

supersonic having a speed greater than the speed of sound.

supply voltage the voltage required to power electrical equipment or an electronic circuit, specified as an a.c. or a d.c. voltage. In the case of an a.c. voltage, the frequency is also specified.

suppurative discharging pus. As an inflamed wound might be, for example.

supra-aural *see* SUPRA-AURAL EARPHONE.

supra-aural earphone an earphone designed so that the cushion of the earphone sits on top of the pinna. As opposed to a circumaural earphone, where the cushion surrounds the pinna.

supra-threshold above the perceptual threshold. Also known as supraliminal. *See also* SUB-THRESHOLD.

supraliminal *see* SUPRA-THRESHOLD.

suprasegmental speech features features of speech which occur on the timescale of a word or phrase, such as intonation, stress and timing. As opposed to segmental speech features which occur on a shorter timescale. Also known as prosodic features. *See also* PROSODY.

surface acoustic wave (SAW) a particular type of acoustic wave which has significant amplitude within only a few wavelengths of the surface of an elastic medium. Surface waves are characterized by both shear distortion and compression of the medium.

surface wave *see* SURFACE ACOUSTIC WAVE.

surround sound the reproduction of sound such that it appears to come from all sides of the listener, using several (usually four or more) separately driven loudspeakers, appropriately distributed around the listening room. *See also* STEREOPHONIC, QUADRAPHONIC.

sweep frequency *see* SWEEP GENERATOR.

sweep generator a signal generator in which the output frequency can be set to vary continuously with time, repeatedly over a specified range. The output may be referred to as a frequency sweep or a sweep frequency. *See also* FREQUENCY GLIDE.

syllable a unit of speech which consists of one or more phonemes: a vowel on its own or a vowel with one or more consonants. A word consists of one or more syllables; hence the syllable may be considered as an intermediate unit of speech, lying between the phoneme and the word. *See also* MORPHEME.

synaesthesia a condition in which the

stimulation of one sense modality causes an additional 'phantom' perception in a different sense. For example, words or sounds may produce an associated visual perception of colour for the listener. The American spelling is synesthesia.

syndrome a medical condition which is identified by the co-occurrence of a number of different attributes.

synesthesia *see* SYNAESTHESIA.

synthesiser or **synthesizer (in electronics)** a device for generating electronic signals. The term often applies to a device which allows a large number of parameters to be individually specified within a complex output signal. *See also* SPEECH SYNTHESIS.

synthetic sentences sentences used in speech audiometry that are grammatically correct, constructed from 'real' words, but meaningless. Used to ensure that contextual clues do not assist in the recognition of individual words. *See also* NONSENSE.

synthetic speech *see* SPEECH SYNTHESIS.

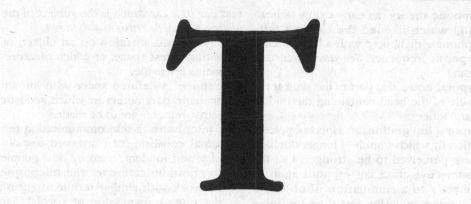

T a switch-position marking found on many hearing aids to indicate the setting in which the input of the hearing-aid amplifier is connected to an induction pick-up coil, in place of the usual microphone, for use with induction loops (which may be fitted around a room) or for inductive coupling to suitable telephones. The letter *T* was chosen because such coils were originally designed for use with telephones. *See also* INDUCTION COIL..

TDD telephone device for deaf people, a term used in the USA for a text telephone.

THD *see* HARMONIC DISTORTION.

TTS *see* TEMPORARY THRESHOLD SHIFT.

tactile aid an aid in which touch stimuli derived from speech (or from other sounds) are used to transmit limited acoustic information to the user. *See also* VIBROTACTILE SENSATION, ELECTRO-TACTILE EFFECT.

tactile sensation a touch sensation, created by small-scale displacement or vibration of the skin. *See also* ELECTROTACTILE EFFECT, VIBROTACTILE SENSATION.

talk-back a facility in a recording studio or an audiometric room which allows a person inside the room to speak to a person outside the room.. The person outside the room may listen either through headphones or a loudspeaker.

talk-forward a facility in a recording studio or an audiometric room which allows an operator outside the room to speak to a person in the room. The person inside the room may listen either through headphones or a loudspeaker.

talk-listen switch for a communication system which allows communication in only one direction at a time, a switch which changes the direction of communication, i.e., determining whether the operator can listen to the person at the other end of the system, or can speak to them.

Tartini tone *see* COMBINATION TONE.

tectorial membrane a soft glutinous membrane which covers the organ of Corti and to which the hair cells are attached on the underside. *See* Figure 2, under EAR.

telephone amplifier an amplifier built into the handset of a telephone to provide additional amplification of the received speech signal before it is sent to the earpiece. An amplifier may also be built into the handset to amplify the speech of a person who cannot produce speech at a normal level.

telephone pick-up coil *see* INDUCTION COIL, T.

telephone theory an early theory of hearing which likened the ear to a telephone switchboard with a line for each specific frequency. *See also* PLACE THEORY.

temporal bone that part of the skull at the side of the head containing the middle and inner ear.

temporal integration an aspect of perception by which stimuli of longer duration are perceived to be stronger, i.e., the subjective effect corresponds approximately to a summation of objective stimulus intensity over time (or, more accurately, over a characteristic time window). For example, as a consequence of temporal integration in the auditory system, the threshold of hearing becomes progressively lower as the duration of test signals is increased from, say, 20 ms to 200 ms.

temporal resolution the ability of a device or a person to distinguish the temporal structure of a signal. Temporal resolution may be evaluated in terms of the fastest timescale on which a signal element such as a gap can be detected. *See also* GAP DETECTION.

temporary threshold shift (TTS) a reversible increase in hearing threshold resulting from exposure to high-level sound. After the high-level sound has ceased, the threshold usually returns to normal over a timescale ranging from minutes to hours, depending on the amount of the preceding sound exposure. *See also* PERMANENT THRESHOLD SHIFT – a similar phenomenon whose effects are long term.

tensor tympani a small muscle attached to the eardrum via the foot of the malleus which is activated by loud sound so as to reduce somewhat the efficiency of sound transmission through the middle ear. *See* Figure 2, under EAR.

test battery an assembly of different tests; for example, to assess a variety of aspects of a hearing impairment.

test box *see* ACOUSTIC TEST BOX.

test ear the ear which is the subject of the test signal. *See also* NON-TEST EAR.

test point the position on an object, or within a test space, at which measurements are made.

test space a defined space with known acoustic parameters in which acoustic measurements are to be made.

text telephone a telecommunication terminal, consisting of a keyboard, text display and modem, used by deaf people to communicate over the telephone network with similar terminals (using the same transmission protocols). *See also* BAUDOT.

thermal noise in electronics, a noise signal produced by the random movement of electrons within a circuit. Also known as Johnson noise. *See also* INHERENT NOISE, SHOT NOISE.

third-octave analysis analysis of a signal by decomposing it into adjacent third-octave bands. *See also* OCTAVE-BAND ANALYSIS, THIRD-OCTAVE FILTER.

third-octave band (1) a range of frequency whose upper and lower limits are separated by one third of an octave.

third-octave band (2) a signal with a bandwidth of one third of an octave.

third-octave filter a bandpass filter whose bandwidth is one third of an octave, i.e., for which the ratio of the upper band-edge frequency to the lower band-edge frequency is 1.26:1. A set of third-octave filters covering adjacent frequency ranges can be used for spectrum analysis. Standardized centre frequencies for such third-octave filters are specified in IEC 61260. *See also* BAND PASS FILTER.

threshold *see* DETECTION THRESHOLD, DISCRIMINATION THRESHOLD, SPEECH-INTELLIGIBILITY THRESHOLD, THRESHOLD OF HEARING, THRESHOLD OF PAIN.

threshold of audibility an alternative term, little used, for threshold of hearing.

threshold of discomfort *see* LOUDNESS DISCOMFORT LEVEL.

threshold of hearing for a given listener, the minimum sound pressure level of a specified sound that is capable of evoking an auditory sensation. The sound reaching the ears from other sources is assumed to be negligible. *Note*: The general conditions of the measurement are to be specified – listening by one ear, two ears, in free field, with earphones, method of constant stimuli or with interrupted sounds, number of trials, etc. (IEC 801-29-18). Also known as hearing threshold. *See also* DETECTION THRESHOLD, NORMAL THRESHOLD OF HEARING, SPEECH DETECTION THRESHOLD LEVEL.

threshold of pain (in electroacoustics) for a given listener, the minimum sound pressure level of a specified sound that will stimulate the ear to a sensation of definite pain. *Note*: The conditions of the measurement are to be specified, similarly to the threshold of hearing (IEC 801-29-23). *See also* NORMAL THRESHOLD OF PAIN.

threshold shift a change (usually an increase) in hearing threshold between measurements on two separate occasions. *See also* TEMPORARY THRESHOLD SHIFT.

throat microphone a microphone worn on the throat, designed to pick up sounds and vibrations which emanate from the throat region when the wearer is speaking. Used in high-noise environments.

tie-clip microphone *see* LAPEL MICROPHONE, LAVALIERE MICROPHONE.

timbre that attribute of auditory sensation which enables a listener to judge that two non-identical sounds having the same loudness and pitch are dissimilar. *Note*: Timbre depends primarily upon the waveform, but also upon the sound pressure and the temporal characteristics of the sound. (IEC 801-29-09).

time-average sound level *see* EQUIVALENT CONTINUOUS SOUND PRESSURE LEVEL.

time-average sound pressure level *see* EQUIVALENT CONTINUOUS SOUND PRESSURE LEVEL.

time constant the characteristic response time of a system, for example, of an AGC circuit. The term is particularly used in connection with systems having an exponential time response, in which case the following definition (IEC 801-21-45) is appropriate: The time required for the amplitude of that component of a field quantity which decays exponentially with time to change by the factor $1/e = 0.3679$. *See also* ATTACK TIME, DECAY TIME, RELEASE TIME, RISE TIME.

time weighting (1) in a sound level meter, the process of time averaging used to obtain the time-mean-square value of the acoustic pressure.

time weighting (2) a descriptor indicating the time constant of the time-averaging circuitry in a sound level meter, standardised as 'F' for fast, 'S' for slow or 'I' for impulse. The time constant for 'F' is 125 ms and for 'S' is 1000 ms; for 'I' the attack time is 35 ms and the decay time is 1500 ms. The characteristics are specified in IEC 651 Sound Level Meters. *See also* INTEGRATION TIME.

tinnitus the sensation of sound experienced by an individual when there is no external acoustic signal present. The perceived sound, which is often a high-pitched whistle or a rushing noise, may appear to be in either ear, in both ears or in the centre of the head. The sensation is generally of neural origin, but may sometimes derive from internally generated sound or vibration in or near the ear, in which case the term objective tinnitus is used. *See also* PHYSIOLOGICAL NOISE, RESIDUAL INHIBITION, TINNITUS MASKER.

tinnitus masker a device, often worn like a hearing aid, which produces a noise in the ear of the user, intended to mask tinnitus. Also known simply as a masker.

tomography *see* X-RAY CT.

tone (1) a sound with a frequency content such that a definite pitch can be ascribed by a listener. A pure tone is a sound with only a single frequency component, i.e., a sinewave.

tone (2) an interval used in conventional Western music. On many musical instruments the tone is standardized as an equally-tempered tone, corresponding to a fundamental-frequency ratio of the sixth root of two. *See also* EQUALLY TEMPERED SCALE.

tone burst a short-duration tone, often a short-duration sinewave. *See also* BRIEF TONE.

tone control a control which changes the frequency response of an audio amplifier, e.g., to increase/decrease the output at low frequencies or increase/decrease the output at high frequencies. *See also* BASS BOOST, BASS CUT, HIGH-FREQUENCY BOOST, HIGH-FREQUENCY CUT.

tone-corrected perceived noise level *see* PERCEIVED NOISE LEVEL.

tone deaf a term used to describe a person who has poor perception of musical pitch and/or little ability to sing in tune.

tone decay a reduction with time in the perceived loudness of a sustained tone whose measured level remains constant. *See also* ADAPTATION.

tone pip *see* brief tone.

total communication a term indicating that both spoken language and sign language are used together in interpersonal communication, used mainly to describe a strategy for the education of deaf children. *See also* ORALISM.

total deafness the condition of having no measurable hearing, i.e., no auditory response when measured with an audiometer capable of providing outputs up to 120 dB HL.

total harmonic distortion *see* HARMONIC DISTORTION.

toy test an audiometric procedure for young children in which the child responds by moving a toy when a test signal is detected. *See also* CONDITIONING, GO GAME, PLAY AUDIOMETRY, VISUAL-REINFORCEMENT AUDIOMETRY.

tragus a small projection of cartilage in front of the opening of the ear canal, part of the external ear; the antitragus is a similar projection on the opposite side of the opening. *See* Figure 2, under EAR.

transducer a device designed to receive an input signal of a given kind and to provide an output signal of a different kind, in such a manner that desired characteristics of the input signal appear in the output signal (IEC 801-25-04). A microphone is an example of a transducer: it receives an acoustic input and produces a corresponding electrical output; similarly, a loudspeaker is a transducer which receives an electrical input and produces a corresponding acoustic output. *See also* ACTIVE TRANSDUCER, ELECTROACOUSTIC TRANSDUCER, ELECTROMECHANICAL TRANSDUCER.

transfer function a description of the change in a sinewave signal as it passes from the input to the output of a device or system. The change in amplitude and the change in phase are given as a function of the signal frequency, either graphically or by means of a mathematical expression. Thus the transfer function incorporates information on both the frequency response and the phase response.

transient (1) a signal or signal component exhibiting a significant change over a short period of time, generally in an otherwise steady or slowly changing context.

transient (2) the response of a system to a sudden disturbance in input conditions, generally decaying with time after the change in input.

transmission loss the reduction in sound pressure level between two designated locations in a sound transmission system, one location often being at a reference distance from the source (IEC 801-23-39). *See also* SOUND INSULATION.

transposition *see* FREQUENCY TRANSPOSITION.

transverse wave a wave in which the direction of particle displacement at each point of the medium is parallel to the wavefront (IEC 801-23-09), i.e., normal to the direction of wave propagation. *See also* LONGITUDINAL WAVE.

trauma *see* ACOUSTIC TRAUMA.

travelling wave a progressive wave: a wave in which the oscillation progresses through space. *See also* STANDING WAVE.

Treacher-Collins syndrome a condition which involves a misshapen head and face with the outer ear and ear canal often missing or very distorted.

tremolo a tonal effect in music that depends primarily on a periodic variation of the amplitude of the sound, at a rate of 5 Hz or so. *See also* VIBRATO.

triangular wave a signal whose waveform consists of repeated sections, each with a linear rise followed by a similar linear fall. *See also* SINEWAVE, SAWTOOTH WAVE, SQUARE WAVE.

trochee a two-syllable word with the first syllable stressed and the second unstressed, for example, 'badger'. Single words used for measurement of speech recognition are generally chosen as monosyllables, spondees or trochees.

Tullio phenomenon dizziness or loss of balance brought on by the presence of loud sound.

tuning fork a two-pronged steel fork designed to produce, when struck, a pure-tone sound wave of specific frequency.

tuning-fork tests simple tests of hearing, now largely superseded by electro-acoustic methods, in which the acoustic stimulus is provided by a tuning fork. *See also* BING TEST, RINNE TEST, WEBER TEST.

tweeter a small loudspeaker designed to operate over the high-frequency part of the audible range. *See also* WOOFER.

two-cc coupler (often written as **2 cc coupler**) a colloquial reference to the acoustic coupler specified in IEC 126 for measurement of the acoustic output of hearing-aid insert earphones. The coupler has a cavity of approximately two cubic centimetres in front of the measuring microphone, hence '2 cc'. *See also* ACOUSTIC COUPLER.

tympanic membrane *see* EARDRUM.

tympanogram the result of tympanometry: a plot of the impedance of the middle ear with changes in the air pressure in the ear canal. The measurement is normally reported in terms of an equivalent volume (i.e., the volume of air whose acoustic impedance has the same magnitude as that measured in the ear), or in terms of the acoustic compliance of this equivalent volume.

tympanometry an audiometric procedure for measuring the acoustic impedance of the middle ear, allowing abnormal conditions to be identified. An acoustic signal is introduced into the sealed external auditory canal and its reflection from the eardrum is monitored. Measurements may be made as a function of the static air pressure in the auditory canal, this pressure being varied by use of a small pump. The measurement is normally reported in terms of an equivalent volume (i.e., the volume of air whose acoustic impedance has the same magnitude as that measured in the ear), or in terms of the acoustic compliance of this equivalent volume. Also known as acoustic-impedance audiometry, immittance audiometry.

tympanoplasty the operation to repair perforations in the eardrum.

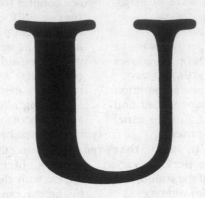

ULL uncomfortable listening level. *See* LOUDNESS DISCOMFORT LEVEL.

ultrasonic relating to ultrasound; above the high-frequency limit of audible sound (around 16 kHz).

ultrasound an acoustic oscillation whose frequency is above the high-frequency limit of audible sound (about 16 kHz) (IEC 801-21-04). *See also* INFRASOUND.

uncomfortable listening level (ULL) *see* LOUDNESS DISCOMFORT LEVEL.

unidirectional microphone a directional microphone the response of which has a prominent maximum for one direction of the sound wave (IEC 801-26-07). Usually a microphone which has a greater sensitivity to sound coming directly towards the front of the microphone rather than from any other angle. *See also* DIRECTIONAL MICROPHONE, OMNIDIRECTIONAL.

unilateral on one side. For example, a unilateral hearing loss is one which occurs in one ear only. *See also* BILATERAL.

unipolar pulse *see* MONOPHASIC PULSE.

unoccluded ear an ear which has no covering or blockage to prevent the entry of sound into the ear canal.

unvoiced *see* VOICED.

Usher's syndrome *see* RETINITIS PIGMENTOSA.

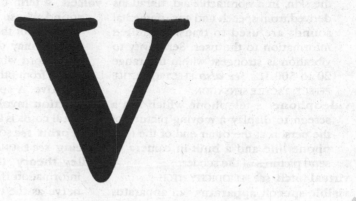

VIIth nerve *see* FACIAL NERVE.

VIIIth nerve *see* AUDITORY NERVE.

VOT *see* VOICE ONSET TIME.

VRA *see* VISUAL-REINFORCEMENT AUDIOMETRY.

VU meter a meter for measuring the level of time-varying signals such as speech or music, widely used in audio equipment and specified for speech audiometers. The time constant of the measurement system is 65 ms, intended to approximate to the time response of the human ear. The characteristics of such a meter are specified in IEC 60268-17. *See also* PEAK PROGRAMME METER.

variable-reluctance loudspeaker *see* ELECTROMAGNETIC LOUDSPEAKER.

variable-reluctance microphone *see* ELECTROMAGNETIC MICROPHONE.

vector quantity a quantity that is characterized by a magnitude and a direction, such as force, velocity, etc. (as opposed to a scalar quantity, such as mass, which is completely characterized by its magnitude).

Velotype a commercially available computer-aided shorthand system in which an operator types on a purpose-designed phonemic keyboard to make verbatim transcriptions of meetings, conferences, etc. Used to provide real-time transcriptions for deaf people. Similar to the computer-aided versions

of the Stenotype and Palantype systems.

vented earmould *see* EARMOULD.

vestibular function the function of the vestibular system, providing the sense of balance.

vestibular system the organ of balance, part of the inner ear, composed of the three semicircular canals, their contents and associated neural systems. *See* Figure 2, under EAR.

vibrating pillow a device used by deaf people to alert them to the presence of alarm signals while in bed, often connected to a special alarm clock.

vibration meter an apparatus for the measurement of the displacement, velocity, or acceleration of a vibrating body (IEC 801-28-15).

vibrato a family of tonal effects in music that depend on periodic variations of one or more characteristics of a sound wave such as frequency and phase, and amplitude, at a rate in the vicinity of six hertz (IEC 801-30-05). *See also* TREMOLO.

vibrator a device for inducing mechanical vibration into an object. *See also* BONE VIBRATOR, VIBRATING PILLOW.

vibrotactile aid *see* VIBROTACTILE SENSATION.

vibrotactile sensation a touch sensation induced by a vibration at the surface of the skin. In a vibrotactile aid, vibrations derived from speech and environmental sounds are used to transmit limited information to the user. Sensitivity to vibration is strongest within the range 20 to 500 Hz. *See also* ELECTROTACTILE EFFECT, TACTILE SENSATION.

videophone a telephone which has a screen to display a moving picture of the person at the other end of the telephone line and a built-in camera to send pictures of the sender.

virtual pitch *see* PERIODICITY PITCH.

visible-speech apparatus an apparatus that displays a spectrum of speech as a function of time. The apparatus may be used to yield a visible portrayal of speech and hence can aid recognition of voice sounds (IEC 801-28-19). In other words, a sound spectrograph operating in real time.

visual-reinforcement audiometry (VRA) a form of audiometry, mainly used with young children, in which a pleasing picture is displayed to the child when he/she responds appropriately. *See also* CONDITIONING, GO GAME, PLAY AUDIOMETRY, TOY TEST.

vocal cords the folds of membrane in the throat, more specifically in the larynx (voicebox), that vibrate to produce the voiced sounds of speech.

vocal tract the acoustic system formed by the cavities in the throat, mouth and nose which act as resonators in the production of speech sounds.

vocalization *see* PHONATION.

vocoder an apparatus for analysis of speech signals in terms of the response of a multiply resonant system to various excitations, followed by the corresponding re-synthesis of the speech from the appropriate excitation and resonance data. The name derives from 'voice coder'.

voice onset time (VOT) the time interval between the release of a stop (plosive) and the onset of the subsequent voicing.

voice simulator *see* ARTIFICIAL VOICE.

voicebox *see* LARYNX.

voiced a term used to describe a speech sound whose production involves the vibration of the vocal cords. The sound energy may derive entirely from the vocal-cord vibration, as in a vowel, or partly from other sources, as in a voiced fricative. A speech sound whose production involves no vibration of the vocal cords is known as unvoiced.

voiceprint *see* SOUND SPECTROGRAPH.

voicing *see* PHONATION, VOICED.

volley theory the theory that frequency information is conveyed in the auditory nerve as the temporal pattern of neurone firing.

voltage sensitivity *see* PRESSURE SENSITIVITY.

volume acceleration for sound travelling in a pipe, for example, the time differential of the volume velocity, i.e., the product of the particle acceleration associated with the sound wave and the cross-sectional area through which the wave is passing.

volume control a manual control of the gain of an amplifier, used to adjust the acoustic output. Sometimes called the gain control.

volume displacement for sound travelling in a pipe, for example, the product of the particle displacement associated with the sound wave and the cross-sectional area through which the wave is passing.

volume velocity for sound travelling in a pipe, for example, the time differential of the volume displacement, i.e., the product of the particle velocity associated with the sound wave and the cross-sectional area through which the wave is passing.

vowel a voiced speech sound of relatively high intensity and length, in English most often occurring between two consonants. English vowels may be divided into two classes: short and long. An example of the former is the sound *i* in 'hid'; an example of the latter is the sound *ee* in 'heed'. *See also* DIPHTHONG, FORMANT.

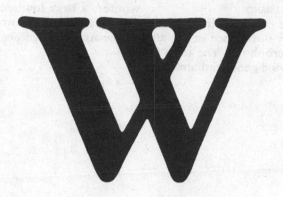

WHO World Health Organization.

Waardenburg's syndrome a condition which involves hearing loss associated with eyes of different colours and a white streak in the hair at the forehead.

warble tone a sound whose frequency varies periodically about a mean value (IEC 801-21-07). A frequency modulated sinewave used for sound-field audiometry. A warble tone covers a band of frequencies (as opposed to an unmodulated sinewave at a single frequency only) and thus offers advantages when used in acoustic environments which may have relatively sharp resonant peaks.

wave the means by which a physical disturbance is transmitted through a medium, without the medium itself being transported. *See also* TRAVELLING WAVE, STANDING WAVE.

waveform the 'shape' of a signal, i.e., the instantaneous magnitude plotted as a function of time. As viewed on an oscilloscope, for example.

wax *see* CERUMEN.

Weber's law states that, for a particular sensory modality and a particular stimulus parameter, the just-noticeable difference (JND) in the stimulus parameter is proportional to the magnitude of that parameter. For example, for an acoustic signal, the JND in intensity is proportional to the intensity at which the JND measurement is carried out.

Weber test a bone-conduction test, often performed with a tuning fork, to investigate a possible unilateral conductive hearing loss. *See also* BING TEST, RINNE TEST, TUNING-FORK TESTS.

weighted sound pressure level *see* SOUND LEVEL.

weighting *see* FREQUENCY WEIGHTING, TIME WEIGHTING.

weighting network an electronic circuit that sets the frequency response or time response of an instrument such as a sound level meter. *See also* FREQUENCY WEIGHTING, TIME WEIGHTING.

whisper test a test in which the tester produces whispered speech to determine the hearing ability of an individual. The test is not normally considered reliable, due to the inherent variability in generating whispered speech and to the wide range of hearing losses which it is necessary to diagnose.

white noise noise whose power spectral density is essentially independent of frequency (IEC 801-21-10), i.e., with a flat power spectrum. An acoustic white-noise signal has the characteristics of a continuous 'rushing' sound. *See also* PINK NOISE.

wideband *see* BROADBAND.

wind noise noise produced in a microphone signal by turbulence in the air around the microphone. The term is also used for wind-generated ambient noise.

woofer a large loudspeaker designed to operate over the low-frequency part of the audible range. *See also* TWEETER.

XYZ

X-ray CT X-ray computed tomography. A method of radiography based on imaging the subject from many directions, providing data that can be used to visualize a selected plane within the body.

Y lead an earphone lead in which one connection from an output socket branches into two connections to two separate earphones.

zero-beat condition *see* BEAT.

zero crossing in a time-varying signal, the event when the signal moves through zero, i.e., its value changes from positive to negative, or vice versa.

zero-crossing frequency for a time-varying signal whose polarity is continuously changing (positive to negative, then negative to positive, etc.), the frequency with which the signal moves through zero, normally taken as the number of positive to negative crossings per second or (equivalently) the number of negative to positive crossings per second.

zero error *see* OFFSET ERROR.

zero level the reference value for a quantity which is expressed in decibels or similar logarithmic units. So called because logarithmic conversion of a value equal to the reference value will give a level of zero.

Zwislocki coupler an artificial ear for the measurement of the sound pressure produced by an insert earphone. Named after the designer J. Zwislocki who provided the basis for the development of the IEC occluded ear simulator, specified in IEC 711.

Appendix 1
Standards relevant to hearing and acoustics

The following table lists the standards cited in the dictionary together with other relevant standards. Standards are listed in terms of their international numbers where relevant. European and national standards that derive from these standards will normally carry the same numbers but have a prefix, for example IEC 60645-1 which is adopted as a British standard and is also a European standard is numbered as BS EN 60645-1.

Due to the significant change in numbers of some standards, particularly in IEC, the older or current number is listed under 'Number' and then the new number is given where appropriate. The current titles are given. Dates are not given for the publications and readers are advised to check for the latest versions.

The list is not comprehensive but does contain those standards considered to be most relevant. Readers should consult their national standards organization for copies of standards and for further information. Comprehensive information on IEC and ISO standards can be obtained from their respective web sites at **www.iec.ch** and **www.iso.ch** .

Number	New Number	Title
BS 0 Part 1	–	A standard for standards Part 1. Context, aims and general principles.
BS 4198	–	Method for calculating loudness.
BS 4727 Part 1	–	British Standard Glossary of electrotechnical power, telecommunication, electronics, lighting and colour terms Part 1 Terms common to power, telecommunications and electronics. Group 04. Measurement terminology.
CD-ROM DICT.	–	1999 IEC Multilingual Dictionary – Electricity, Electronics and Telecommunications.
IEC 50(801)	IEC 60050-801	International Electrotechnical Vocabulary Chapter 801: Acoustics and electroacoustics.
IEC 118-0	IEC 60118-0	Hearing aids Part 0: Measurement of electroacoustical characteristics.
IEC 118-1	IEC 60118-1	Hearing aids Part 1: Hearing aids with induction pick-up coil input.
IEC 118-2	IEC 60118-2	Hearing aids Part 2: Hearing aids with automatic gain control circuits.

IEC 118-3	IEC 60118-3	Hearing aids Part 3: Hearing aid equipment not entirely worn on the body.
IEC 118-4	IEC 60118-4	Hearing aids Part 4: Magnetic field strength in audio-frequency induction loops for hearing aid purposes.
IEC 118-5	IEC 60118-5	Hearing aids Part 5: Nipples for insert earphones.
IEC 118-6	IEC 60118-6	Hearing aids Part 6: Characteristics of electrical input circuits for hearing aids.
IEC 118-7	IEC 60118-7	Hearing aids Part 7: Measurement of the performance characteristics of hearing aids for quality inspection for delivery purposes.
IEC 118-8	IEC 60118-8	Hearing aids Part 8: Methods of measurement of perform-ance characteristics of hearing aids under simulated in situ working conditions.
IEC 118-9	IEC 60118-9	Hearing aids Part 9: Methods of measurement of characteristics of hearing aids with bone vibrator outputs.
IEC 118-10	IEC 60118-10	Hearing aids Part 10: Guide to hearing aid standards.
IEC 118-11	IEC 60118-11	Hearing aids Part 11: Symbols and other markings on hearing aids and related equipment.
IEC 118-12	IEC 60118-12	Hearing aids Part 12: Dimensions of electrical connector systems.
IEC 118-13	IEC 60118-13	Hearing aids Part 13: Electromagnetic compatibility (EMC).
–	IEC 60118-14	Hearing aids Part 14: Specification of a digital interface device.
IEC 268-2	IEC 60268-2	Sound system equipment Part 2: Explanation of general terms and calculation methods.
IEC 268-10	IEC 60268-10	Sound system equipment Part 10: Peak programme level meters.
IEC 268-17	IEC 60268-17	Sound system equipment Part 17: Standard volume indicators.
IEC 318	IEC 60318-1	Electroacoustics – Simulators of human head and ear – Part 1: Ear simulator for the calibration of supra-aural earphones.
IEC 60050-891	–	International Electrotechnical Vocabulary – Part 891: Electrobiology.
IEC 60318-2	–	Electroacoustics – Simulators of human head and ear – Part 2: An interim acoustic coupler for the calibration of audiometric earphones in the high frequency range.
IEC 303	IEC 60318-3	Electroacoustics – Simulators of human head and ear – Part 3: Acoustic coupler for the calibration of supra-aural

Number	New Number	Title
		earphones used in audiometry.
IEC 711	IEC 60318-4	Electroacoustics – Simulators of human head and ear – Part 4: Occluded ear simulator for the measurement of earphones coupled to the ear by ear inserts.
IEC 126	IEC 60318-5	Electroacoustics – Simulators of human head and ear – Part 5: IEC reference coupler for the measurement of hearing aids using earphones coupled to the ear by ear inserts.
IEC 373	IEC 60318-6	Electroacoustics – Simulators of human head and ear – Part 6: Mechanical coupler for measurements on bone vibrators.
IEC 645-1	IEC 60645-1	Audiometers – Part 1: Pure tone audiometers.
IEC 645-2	IEC 60645-2	Audiometers – Part 2: Equipment for speech audiometry.
IEC 645-3	IEC 60645-3	Audiometers – Part 3: Auditory test signals of short duration for audiometric and neuro-otological purposes.
IEC 645-4	IEC 60645-4	Audiometers – Part 4: Equipment for extended high-frequency audiometry.
IEC 651	–	Sound level meters
IEC 60942	–	Electroacoustics – Sound calibrators.
IEC 804	IEC 6084	Integrating-averaging sound level meters.
IEC/TR 959	IEC/TR 60959	Provisional head and torso simulator for acoustic measurements on air conduction hearing aids.
IEC 1027	IEC 61027	Instruments for the measurement of aural acoustic impedance/admittance.
IEC 1260	IEC 61260	Electroacoustics – Octave-band and fractional octave-band filters.
IEC 61252	–	Electroacoustics – Specifications for personal sound exposure meters.
ISO 16	–	Acoustics – Standard tuning frequency (Standard musical pitch).
ISO 389	ISO 389-1	Reference zero for the calibration of audiometric equipment – Part 1: Reference equivalent threshold sound pressure levels for pure tones and supra-aural earphones.
	ISO 389-2	Reference zero for the calibration of audiometric equipment – Part 2: Reference equivalent sound pressure levels for pure tones and insert earphones.
	ISO 389-3	Reference zero for the calibration of audiometric equipment – Part 3: Reference equivalent threshold force levels for pure tones and bone vibrators.
	ISO 389-4	Reference zero for the calibration of audiometric

Number	New Number	Title
		equipment – Part 4: Reference levels for narrow-band masking.
	ISO/TR 389-5	Reference zero for the calibration of audiometric equipment – Part 5: Reference equivalent threshold sound pressure levels for pure tones in the frequency range 8 kHz to 16 kHz.
ISO 226	ISO 389-7	Reference zero for the calibration of audiometric equipment – Part 7: Reference threshold of hearing under free-field and diffuse-field listening conditions.
ISO 266	–	Acoustics – Preferred frequencies for measurements.
ISO/R 532	–	Acoustics – Methods for calculating loudness.
ISO 1683	–	Preferred reference quantities for acoustic levels.
ISO 1999	–	Acoustics – Determination of occupational noise exposure and estimation of noise-induced hearing impairment.
ISO 3891	–	Acoustics – Procedures for describing aircraft noise heard on the ground.
ISO 4869-1	–	Acoustics – Hearing protectors – Part 1: Subjective method for the measurement of sound attenuation.
ISO 4869-2	–	Acoustics – Hearing protectors – Part 2: Estimation of effective A-weighted sound pressure levels when hearing protectors are worn.
ISO 4869-3	–	Acoustics – Hearing protectors – Part 3: Simplified method for the measurement of insertion loss of ear-muff type protectors for quality inspection purposes.
ISO 4869-4	–	Acoustics – Hearing protectors Part 4: Methods for the measurement of sound attenuation of amplitude-sensitive hearing protectors.
ISO 6189	–	Acoustics – Pure tone air conduction audiometry for hearing conservation purposes.
ISO 7029	–	Acoustics – Statistical distribution of hearing thresholds as a function of age.
ISO 8253-1	–	Acoustics – Audiometric test methods – Part 1: Basic pure tone air and bone conduction audiometry.
ISO 8253-2	–	Acoustics – Audiometric test methods – Part 2: Sound field audiometry with pure tone and narrow-band test signals.
ISO 8253-3	–	Acoustics – Audiometric test methods – Part 3: Speech audiometry.
ISO 9999	–	Technical aids for disabled persons – Classification.

References

Brinkmann K, Richter U (1997) Ensuring reliability and comparability of speech audiometry in Germany. In: M. Martin (Ed) Speech Audiometry. Whurr Publishers, London.

BSA (1998) British Society of Audiology recommendation: Descriptors for pure-tone audiograms. British Journal of Audiology 22, 123.

BSA (1975) British Society of Audiology: Standard Forms for Results of Audiometry. British Journal of Audiology 9, yellow pages.

Carhart R (1951) Basic principles of speech audiometry. Acta Otolaryngologica 40: 62–71.

WHO (1980) International Classification of Impairments, Disabilities and Handicaps. Geneva: World Health Organisation, pp. 31, 45.